Nature's Pharmacy for Children

Drug-free Alternatives for More Than 200 Childhood Ailments

Lendon H. Smith, M.D.

Lynne Paige Walker, Pharm.D., MCTM, Homo.D., LAC, Rph

Ellen Hodgson Brown, J.D.

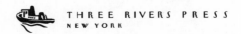

THREE RIVERS PRESS
NEW YORK

This book should only be used as a reference in an ongoing partnership between doctor and patient (or patient's parent). It is not a substitute for your doctor's professional judgment and is intended only to raise issues for discussion with a physician before embarking on or terminating any form of treatment.

Published by Three Rivers Press, New York, New York.
Member of the Crown Publishing Group.

Random House, Inc. New York, Toronto, London, Sydney, Auckland
www.randomhouse.com

THREE RIVERS PRESS and the Tugboat design are
registered trademarks of Random House, Inc.

Printed in the United States of America

Design by Jo Anne Metsch

Library of Congress Cataloging-in-Publication Data
Smith, Lendon H., 1921–
Nature's pharmacy for children : drug-free alternatives for more than
200 childhood ailments / by Lendon H. Smith, Lynne Paige Walker,
and Ellen Hodgson Brown.
p. cm.
1. Children—Diseases—Alternative treatment. 2. Naturopathy. 3. Pediatrics.
I. Walker, Lynne Paige. II. Brown, Ellen Hodgson. III. Title.
RJ61 .S6629 2002
615.5'35083—dc21   2001034068

ISBN 0-609-80664-5

10 9 8 7 6 5 4 3 2 1

First Edition

NATURE'S

Acknowledgments

The authors wish to acknowledge the many patients, friends, and relatives who have shared their beneficial results when they switched to a natural body-supporting approach to their own and their children's ailments.

Special thanks to Kathy Arnos for sharing her extensive knowledge of children's ailments and their natural treatment, and to Linda Forbes for her illuminating insights over two decades into the marvelous workings of the body.

Special thanks also to our agent and friend Bob Silverstein of Quicksilver Books for his invaluable aid and advice with this and other projects over the years, and to Sarah Silbert of Crown Books for her astute and efficient editorial help.

Contents

Preface

THIS BOOK brings you the expertise of three recognized authorities in the field of alternative health care and childhood disease. Their combined insights form the basis for a definitive guide designed to give parents choices in managing the ordinary illnesses of their children, without reliance on toxic drugs that suppress natural functions.

Lendon Smith, M.D., has fifty years' experience as a pediatrician and has written sixteen books in the field, including the best-selling *Feed Your Kids Right*. He has been a leader in a growing movement away from the conventional drug approach that attributes disease to genetic and other factors beyond an individual's control. Dr. Smith takes a natural, body-supporting approach: Look for underlying causes; correct nutritional and lifestyle problems; treat by encouraging rather than suppressing the normal cleansing mechanisms of the body.

Dr. Smith modified his pediatric approach after realizing that his medical school curriculum had been underwritten by the pharmaceutical industry. Understanding that medical research and medical journals were financed by drug companies, he began a search for better answers. A chiropractic college and a naturopathic medical school helped him overcome some prejudices acquired in conventional medical school. He advises parents to pay attention to possible dietary and lifestyle factors when their children are sick; find a well-trained medical doctor they can trust; get a diagnosis and a treatment plan; then do some research to find alternative or complementary methods that will resolve their child's health problems safely and inexpensively.

Dr. Lynne Walker is also trained in both the conventional and alternative approaches to disease. Her unique expertise is in the field of remedies. Her first doctorate was in pharmacy; but after working for a number of years as a hospital pharmacist, she became aware of the limitations of pharmaceuticals. Feeling she could no longer recommend them to patients, she went on to obtain doctorates in Chinese medicine and homeopathy. Her experience includes ten years as a hospital pharmacist; five years as pharmacist at the largest and busiest homeopathic pharmacy in the country, Capitol Drugs; fourteen years in private practice as homeopath and acupuncturist; and six years as proprietor of herb companies in Idaho, New York, and California. As a result of this varied experience, she has seen the effects and side effects of drugs and the benefits of a broad range of natural remedies in virtually all of the ailments discussed in the following pages. She has coauthored three books with Ellen Brown, including the best-selling *Nature's Pharmacy*.

Ellen Brown's expertise is in research and writing. She practiced for ten years as an attorney in Los Angeles before switching her focus to medical research. She has written eight books and numerous articles in the field of alternative health care. She brings a particular interest to children's diseases from her own experience as a mother. She recognized the value of a good book when her children were small and suffered from one ear infection after another. They seemed to be continually on antibiotics, causing her to question whether these drugs were doing any good. Her suspicions were confirmed by a book that warned mothers of the hazards of antibiotics and advised them to resist giving the drugs except in certain narrow circumstances. She followed this advice, which proved invaluable. For both of her children, there was a "healing crisis"—a single traumatic episode of the condition—after which they never suffered from ear infections again.

In this book, the authors hope to help other parents gain the confidence to break the drug cycle for their children's common health conditions. The book guides parents through the maze of controversy involving conventional and alternative medical approaches and assists in selecting the best options. In addition to being a handy guide for home treatment of common complaints, the book can help parents speak intelligently to their doctors to get appropriate information and treatment for their families. The discussion is liberally supported throughout with research and case histories taken from the authors' extensive experience with children's ailments.

Remedies and dosages are specifically tempered for the common ailments of children and their smaller bodies, suitable for their finicky tastes and lesser ability to swallow pills. The authors identify products by brand names, naming those that are not only effective but appealing and ingestible for kids. Certain companies are mentioned frequently, not because the authors have stock in the company (they don't) but because these products are easily obtainable throughout the United States and are now found even in many pharmacies. Addresses and phone numbers have been omitted, however, because these companies generally prefer that products be obtained through a practitioner, pharmacy, or health food store.

Drawing from and comparing a number of treatment options—drugs, herbs, nutritional supplements, homeopathic remedies, Chinese patent medicines, flower essences, and essential oils—this book provides an eclectic approach to the treatment of your child's illnesses and behavioral problems, allowing you to choose the best, most appropriate, and generally safest therapies. For further information on products, for private consultations, to order products, or to subscribe to a newsletter, see the websites www.alternativepharmacy.com or www.naturespharmacy.tv.

A WORD TO PARENTS FROM
LENDON SMITH, M.D.

Pediatric medicine has changed significantly in the fifty years since I began my practice. Antibiotics and other drugs have proliferated, and the list of recommended childhood immunizations has gotten longer and more comprehensive. Expensive tests are run for every conceivable condition. Parents are bombarded with drug commercials, and pediatricians with drug-company hype. Doctors feel compelled to come up with a prescription for every cough, stomach ailment, and skin eruption seen in the child; yet more children seem to be sick today than ever before. Not only are common ailments like ear infections more frequent, but chronic complaints like asthma, attention deficit disorder, childhood obesity, and diabetes are on the increase. What has gone wrong? My conclusion, after years of research and clinical experience, is that the modern overprocessed junk-food diet, toxins in the environment, and the rush to drugs are largely to blame.

My principal advice to parents is to assume a wait-and-see attitude toward common children's ailments, giving nature a chance to take its course. Illness is merely the body's way of righting imbalances; coughing, sneezing, diarrhea, and vomiting are how it cleans out toxins. Suppressing those cleansing mechanisms with drugs can only drive the offending toxins deeper into the body, where they are likely to trigger chronic ailments that are much harder to cure.

While you are waiting for childhood illnesses to do their cleansing work, there are natural remedies and therapies that can be used to ease your child's discomfort and speed the process of healing. The purpose of this book is to provide parents with a practical, informative guide to children's ailments, their conventional and alternative treatments, and when and how natural remedies should be used on specific conditions.

Should you use an antibiotic or other drug? Let your child sweat it out? Offer some safe nutrients and hope they work? We offer some alternatives with which you can feel comfortable. We have combined our expertise in furnishing the most up-to-date information available on treating children's ailments naturally, without the adverse effects of drugs. We cover disease factors that your pediatrician might have overlooked, including food sensitivities and allergies; toxins in the air, food, and water; genetic tendencies; and emotional stressors. Many standard medical approaches are now known to be ineffective at best and life-threatening at worst. We alert parents to those hazards and suggest safe and effective alternatives.

INTRODUCTION

A Safer Approach to Children's Diseases

PEDIATRICIANS HAVE traditionally been taught in medical school that parents come to them for a drug prescription, and that if no prescription is forthcoming, the parents will find another doctor. This drug-oriented tactic has caused many a prescription to be written where none was necessary; but times are changing. The sought-after pediatrician is becoming the one who takes a conservative approach, recommending drugs only as a last resort.

According to a 1998 study in *The Journal of the American Medical Association,* more than a hundred thousand deaths now occur annually from legal drugs *prescribed and used correctly.*[1] That makes pharmaceutical side effects the fourth leading cause of death, following only heart disease, cancer, and stroke. This problem is of particular concern for children, whose lower body weights make them more susceptible to adverse reactions. Drugs don't address the cause of disease. They simply mask symptoms. They target the coughing, sneezing, fever, and diarrhea we think of as the problem, when in fact these symptoms represent the body's attempt to get rid of the problem—the foreign toxins, microbes, or chemicals that have built up in the tissues. When these reactions are deadened with drugs, the toxins are left to accumulate in the body, resulting in unwanted "side effects" that make the problem worse.

A conservative approach is warranted not just to reduce side effects but because overuse of drugs is now rendering them ineffective. Drugs that were supposed to eradicate infectious disease are now actually being blamed for the spread of disease. An increasing incidence of staph infections, otitis media (middle-ear infection) among children, and sinusitis among adults is blamed on the overuse of broad-spectrum microbial drugs, creating widespread drug resistance and breeding "superbugs" that are immune to antibiotics. Between 1975 and 1990, office visits for middle-ear infection went up a staggering 175 percent.[2] The vaccines given to prevent common childhood diseases may be spreading disease as well. Recent research links them to an increased incidence of asthma, childhood autism, and SIDS (sudden infant death syndrome). Steroids such as cortisone, which act by suppressing the immune system, are other suspects. Over-the-counter hydrocortisone creams commonly used to suppress itching can prevent the immune system from fighting off infection, turning simple surface infections into serious systemic diseases. (See "Immunity," "Immunizations," "Itching.")

A growing disillusionment with pharmaceuticals has prompted a surge of interest in natural remedies. The natural approach to cure recognizes that the body can heal itself, and that most common complaints will go away if the body is left to its own devices. That doesn't mean, however, that parents must sit by idly and listen to their suffering children cry while nature takes its course. Excellent natural, nontoxic remedies are now available that can ease children's symptoms and help their young bodies heal without adverse effects. Remedies that support the body's efforts to repair itself include nutritional supplements, herbs, homeopathic remedies, aromatherapy, and flower essences.

Herbs and Tonics

HERBS HAVE been used for healing throughout recorded history. Many conventional drugs are extracted from plants. Naturopathic doctors maintain that the whole herb is more therapeutic than its isolated ingredients and is less likely to result in side effects. Statistics from the American Association of Poison Control Centers confirm that while drug poisonings kill hundreds of people annually, deaths from herbal medicine are virtually unheard of.[3]

Herbal remedies are available as pills, teas, drops, and distillations of various sorts. One option is aromatherapy, involving distillations of the essential oils of the plant. These oils carry the plant's important information and have been referred to as the "blood" or "life force" of the plant. Gemmotherapy, another form of herbal therapy, is derived from the baby shoots of plants. Gemmotherapies are said to contain more vital life force than other herbal options, and they taste good, so getting kids to take them is not a problem. The usual dosage is once daily, although in severe cases, they can be given two or three times daily. While the label says gemmotherapies are to be used only by people sixteen years and older, they just need to be diluted with water to make them safe for children. The warning is due simply to the high alcohol content of the fluid carrying the remedies. For children under twelve, give ten or fifteen drops in water once or twice a day; older children may take up to fifty drops a day in water.

For most people, herbal remedies are considered quite safe in recommended doses. However, professional advice is still recommended for children and pregnant women, since a few medicinal plants can cause bodily harm when taken in excess. Doses should be diluted for children. Even with these provisos, herbs are far less risky than their pharmaceutical counterparts.[4]

Parents should be aware that many natural remedies work by stimulating the body to do its own housecleaning, and that while toxic substances are being eliminated through the bloodstream, they can make children more tired and cranky than before the remedy was taken. But this reaction soon passes, and the user is boosted into a higher state of well-being. If you think your child is having an allergic or otherwise excessive reaction to an herbal or other oral remedy, have the child stop taking it and drink copious amounts of water. Give him or her a hot bath to alleviate symptoms.

 ## Bach Flower Remedies

EVEN SAFER for children than herbs are Bach flower remedies. Derived from flowers, these vibrational remedies are entirely nontoxic. Unlike conventional medicine, which works chemically, vibrational remedies are said to work on an energetic level to stimulate the body's own healing energy, rather like a tuning fork that sets disharmonious chords back on track.

Dr. Edward Bach, a British physician, categorized thirty-eight flowers, all of which work on different emotions. Walnut, for example, helps during stressful life changes such as moving. Pine helps with feelings of guilt. Star of Bethlehem helps with shock. The combination Rescue Remedy is very effective for relieving stress and irritability. Bach flowers are a great way to treat children for emotional trauma like the first day of school, death of a pet, or fear of exams.

The remedies can be taken in many ways: Put four drops directly under the tongue up to five times daily. Or place a dropperful in water and have the child sip it throughout the day. You can also mix a dropperful with water in a spray bottle and spray in the room to calm fighting children as they inhale it.

Homeopathy

ANOTHER TYPE of vibrational remedy that is very safe for children is homeopathy. Homeopathic remedies consist of minute doses of natural substances—mineral, plant, or animal—that, if given to healthy people in larger doses, would cause the symptoms a patient is experiencing. Where allopathic or conventional medicine suppresses symptoms, homeopathy encourages them, on the theory that they represent the body's attempt to flush out toxins. Homeopathy involves inducing a mild reaction in the body by simulating the larger reaction constituting the disease. The principle is the same as for pharmaceutical vaccination, but vaccines are macromolecules that can induce unwanted side effects. Homeopathic remedies have no side effects because they are dilute—at some strengths so dilute that no molecule of the original substance is likely to be left in solution. Only its vibration remains.

Homeopathy's current renaissance in the United States is due in part to a series of studies that has finally brought scientific credence to its rather unlikely premises. On September 29, 1997, the British medical journal *The Lancet* reported the results of a meta-analysis (a systematic review of a body of research) of eighty-nine blinded, randomized, placebo-controlled clinical trials of homeopathy. It found that the average effect of the homeopathic medicines used in those studies was 2.45 times greater than placebos. For comparative purposes, in a meta-analysis of twenty well-controlled studies of popular antidepressants, the drugs were found to be only 1.3 times as effective as placebos.[5]

Constitutional homeopaths can make profound changes in people with single, high-potency doses of homeopathic remedies given over long periods of time. Many cases are on record in which serious or even fatal illnesses have been reversed and lab values returned to normal in a few months, results that in Western medical practice would have been considered impossible. Treatment is individualized and largely dependent on the practitioner's experience in selecting the correct remedy. An increasingly popular alternative is for users and parents to educate themselves and select their own homeopathic remedies. Combination remedies take a shotgun approach, including a range of likely homeopathic possibilities that helps take the guesswork out of the selection process.

One proviso: It is much easier for a practitioner to treat a problem at the onset. If time is lost in self-treatment with the wrong remedies, the homeopath will have a harder time. Another proviso: Homeopathic remedies given incorrectly *in high potencies* over a period of time can suppress the disease and worsen the condition, as can any remedy given for a long period after symptoms have cleared. Those provisos aside, single remedies in low potency, and combination homeopathic remedies for minor ailments, are quite safe and effective.

When giving homeopathic remedies to children, use only 3x to 30x potencies, nothing higher, unless the remedies have been chosen by an experienced practitioner. The lowest potency, "x," indicates dilution by ten; "c" indicates dilution by one hundred; "m" by one thousand. In homeopathy, which works vibrationally, the highest dilutions are the strongest remedies, since their vibratory levels are higher. Children's systems are very easily affected, so lower potencies are generally quite effective. You don't need the high potencies. Children also respond rapidly, so the remedies needn't be given for long periods. Here are some other stipulations when using homeopathic remedies:

* Give the remedies a minimum of fifteen minutes before or after eating or drinking anything except water. The mouth should be clean and free of food, drink, toothpaste, gum, etc. Avoid camphor, mint, menthol, and eucalyptus products, which can antidote the remedies (render them ineffective), as can coffee, even coffee-flavored ice cream or candy. Never use homeopathic medicine along with steroid drugs, including hydrocortisone creams. Homeopathic remedies encourage the body to regain its original vitality. Steroids work by an opposing mechanism, suppressing the immune system's own efforts.

* Avoid touching homeopathic remedies with the hands. When taking pellets, shake them into the cap of the bottle, then drop them into your child's mouth. They should be kept under the tongue until they dissolve. When giving liquid remedies, let the drops fall from the dropper or bottle into the mouth, taking care not to touch the dropper to the tongue or lips; or put the drops in a sip of water. Have the child try to hold the liquid in the mouth for thirty seconds before swallowing. Wait at least thirty seconds before giving another remedy.

* Store the remedies in a dark place away from perfumes, medications, foods, herbs, strong-smelling substances, and electronic equipment. When you fly, don't let the remedies be x-rayed or put them in your checked luggage, which is often x-rayed. Carry them separately in a small bag and put them on the key tray when you walk through the doorway at the security check. Pick them up on the other side. (If they accidentally go through the machine, they can still be used; they may just be less effective.)

* Be prepared for a slight aggravation of symptoms, which sometimes takes place before the patient feels better. This effect is not only normal but desirable: It indicates the remedy is appropriate and that healing is beginning to occur. Discontinue the remedy when you see improvement in symptoms. Homeopathic remedies exert subtle influences on the system. Their purpose is to encourage the body on its health-building path. When the body is healthy, it no longer needs the remedy. Prolonged use beyond that time may result in a nontoxic aggravation, producing the very symptoms the remedy was being given to eliminate. If that happens, don't worry; the symptoms will disappear when the remedy is discontinued. If symptoms return after the remedy has been stopped, try giving a few more drops. If you're consulting a practitioner, return within two to three weeks to determine whether the remedy is still needed.

Lifestyle Factors: Diet, Exercise, Sleep

TO ENSURE a basic level of health, parents need to feed their kids right and keep junk food to a minimum. (See "Nutrition," "Breast-feeding.") They should also help children reduce stress and get enough sleep, fresh air, sunshine, and exercise. That means frequent breaks from the computer and the TV. If left to their own devices, children will stay up all night. Parents need to enforce a reasonable bedtime. To ensure that sleep is of the high-quality variety that drops into nightly REM, physical and emotional calm and quiet are important.

Harmful toxins should also be reduced in the environment and in foods, which should be as free as possible from pesticides, preservatives, and food coloring. These additives congest the liver (the organ responsible for cleaning the blood), leading to irritability, anger, and depression. If you paint your child's room, or stain the doors or floor, you can often see the effects in a child's behavior. New carpets, beds, and car interiors all contain formaldehydes that are breathed in and exit only after being broken down by the liver. The more toxic chemicals a child is exposed to, the harder it is for the liver to do its work; and the more congested the liver, the more irritable, angry, depressed, and sluggish the child becomes.

If stressors and junk food are kept to a minimum, if nutrient needs are supplied, and if the body's own efforts at cure are supported rather than suppressed, parents can look forward to enjoying happy, healthy children.

 Getting Prepared: Stocking the Basics

HERE ARE some popular herbal and homeopathic remedies that are good to have on hand for emergency first aid and to treat children's ailments like upset stomachs and congestion.

* Trauma or Traumeel ointment: These homeopathic combination ointments can be massaged into sore muscles or sprains to relieve aches and pains. They also come as oral drops, which can be taken along with topical application at the rate of ten drops every fifteen minutes for the first hour, then ten drops four times daily.

* Calendula lotion is an excellent remedy for diaper rash or any skin irritation.

* Calendula tincture is useful for wound cleaning and healing. Put two droppersful in one pint of water to soak or wash a cut or wound. Then wrap the wound with a calendula-soaked dressing. Healing time can be dramatically reduced with this treatment.

* Rescue Remedy: This is by far the most popular Bach flower essence combination. Excellent for relieving stress and irritability, Rescue Remedy can calm an upset child, an irritable teen, a stressed-out mother, even traumatized pets. It is completely safe, even for babies and pregnant women.

* Peppermint oil: A couple of drops in a glass of warm water will heal a stomachache. For headaches, apply peppermint oil directly to the forehead to stimulate prostaglandins, which relieve pain.

* Biting Insects by Molecular Biologicals: A great remedy to prevent insect bites or stop pain and itch after being bitten. It is safe and effective for children and easy to use. Give ten drops three times daily.

* Elderberry extract (liquid) is a strong antiviral and antibacterial remedy. Give twenty to forty drops, three times daily, at the onset of a cold to help relieve symptoms.

* Olive-leaf extract is another effective antiviral and antibacterial remedy that is quite safe and may be used in place of antibiotics.

* Aloe vera gel: This is a popular topical treatment for sunburn, abrasions, and other skin problems.

* Calendula and Hypericum ointment can be a miracle cure on certain types of cold sores or cuts. Used topically, the ointment can heal cold sores in a single day.

* Homeopathic Arnica 6x or 30x tablets: Taken orally, Arnica can stop trauma to the body and soothe sore muscles, aches, and sprains. A product by Boiron called Arnicalm, consisting of Arnica, Bellis, and Ledum, is particularly good for kids. The remedy you need when your child stubs a toe, slams a finger in the door, or drops something on a foot, Arnica is also good for more serious trauma, such as car accidents that might involve injury or whiplash. It should be taken as soon as possible after trauma—two pills every fifteen minutes for the first hour following a severe trauma, then four times daily as needed.

* Tea tree oil: This remedy has a wealth of uses, although it is strong and best used topically on children. Tea tree oil can be used as an antifungal for athlete's foot, and for fingernail or toenail fungus; as a scalp cleanser for problems like dandruff and lice; as a topical remedy for canker sores, cold sores, acne, minor cuts or abrasions, insect bites, rashes, or minor burns. It can also be used for thrush in babies, but professional advice from a naturopathic practitioner should be sought.

* Black ointment: This is a drawing salve that can pull out slivers of glass or splinters that can't otherwise be removed. It has been used successfully, for example, to draw out cactus needles in the foot. The day after its topical application, the needles become red and encapsulated and pop out when touched. Apply twice daily to the problem area.

* Passiflora 6x is a gentle homeopathic remedy for insomnia.

* Ignatia 30x is a homeopathic remedy for unexpected grief, such as when the family dog dies or your teenage daughter's boyfriend breaks up with her.

* Cantharis 6x is a homeopathic remedy that will take the sting out of a burn. Give two pills every fifteen minutes as needed for pain, then three to four times daily to promote healing. Cantharis is also a great homeopathic remedy for a bladder infection: Give two pills every fifteen minutes for one hour, then two every hour to relieve discomfort. Also provide plenty of water. If the problem has not improved in six to eight hours, seek medical advice.

* Homeopathic Gunpowder 6x is good for any type of minor infection, from that of a pierced ear to an abscessed tooth. The remedy pushes out the infection, aiding healing. The dosage is three pills three to four times daily.

* Chamomilla 6x helps calm cranky, irritable children and quells temper tantrums.

* Bacticin drops: These homeopathic drops stimulate the body to fight bacteria. The dosage is ten drops three to five times daily for strep throat, acne, red and inflamed infections, infections with an odor, and deeper infections causing pus formation and drainage.

* ABC drops: A combination of Aconite, Belladonna, and Chamomilla, this homeopathic remedy is quite popular in Europe for colds and earaches. Give at the onset of symptoms.

* Cold and Flu Solution Plus by Dolisos: Given at the onset of cold symptoms, one every fifteen minutes for the first hour, then one pill four times daily, this remedy has been known to knock out a cold in a single day.

An A-to-Z Guide to Common Children's Ailments and Their Best Treatments

THE FOLLOWING guide presents a wide selection of common children's ailments in handy reference form, including an analysis of drug treatments that are currently popular and the natural alternatives available from various disciplines—homeopathy, herbalism, nutrition, flower essences, aromatherapy, and the like. The focus is on remedies reported by parents to actually work.

ABDOMINAL PAIN

THIS COMMON childhood symptom is most often caused by gas moving sideways in the intestines, which will pass of its own accord. Some abdominal "pain" may be merely a ploy to avoid school or chores; a parent can usually determine this from the child's behavior. Other abdominal pains may be real, though associated with emotional factors. Anxiety over tensions at school or at home can bring on a stomachache.

If short-term abdominal pain causes a doubling-up sort of misery in the child, some attention must be paid to it, since there is a remote possibility that it signals a serious medical condition such as appendicitis (inflammation of the appendix), intussusception (the telescoping of one segment of the bowel into another), or volvulus (a twisting and knotting of the bowel). All can put the child into shock. Long-term abdominal pain lasting weeks or months, especially if accompanied by diarrhea or loose bowel movements, could be colitis or Crohn's disease. Consult a pediatrician to eliminate these possibilities. Serious abdominal problems usually produce a very tender abdomen and muscle-guarding action. A good practice is for parents to feel their child's abdomen when cuddling or massaging him in order to become familiar with his reactions when not ill, providing a base for comparison.

Parasitic infection is an often-overlooked possible cause of abdominal pain. Other symptoms besides stomach pain that are clues to parasites include alternating constipation and diarrhea, pain around the navel, tooth-grinding while sleeping, irritable or mean behavior (pinching, punching, biting), and symptoms that are worse around the full or new moon. (See "Parasites.")

 Evaluating Abdominal Pain

IN MAKING an initial evaluation of your child's abdominal pain, consider its location, how often it occurs, and any other symptoms accompanying it. Is it daily or sporadic? Can it be traced to eating particular foods? Here is a breakdown of abdominal pain based on its location:

Mid-abdominal pain (centered around the navel) generally has its source in the small intestines. Pain that comes and goes suggests that the child has intestinal flu and that vomiting and diarrhea are about to begin. Food sensitivities can also produce mid-abdominal pain.

Lower right abdominal pain that is constant for several hours suggests appendicitis. The typical feeling is one of needing a bowel movement, but the pain is not relieved if a bowel movement occurs.

Upper left abdominal pain following a blow to that area raises the possibility (though remote) of a ruptured spleen, requiring medical attention. Call your pediatrician for advice.

Upper right abdominal pain comes from the area where the liver and gallbladder are located. If a child repeatedly complains of pain in this area, consult your pediatrician, who can perform appropriate tests to determine the cause.

Lower left abdominal pain suggests a lower colon problem like constipation. Such abdominal pain may run in the family, but that doesn't necessarily mean it's genetic; it may be because the entire family is eating a low-roughage diet. See "Constipation."

 ## Natural Home Remedies

ABDOMINAL PAIN from an upset stomach, gas, bloating, or overeating can be relieved with peppermint tea made from bags or loose tea. For temporary relief of chronic abdominal pain (as in Crohn's disease), enteric-coated peppermint tablets are very effective. Peppermint also comes as an essential oil good for stomachaches. Place one drop of peppermint oil in warm water and have the child drink it.

Other herbs and herbal teas that are safe and effective natural alternatives for settling the stomach include licorice, ginger, chamomile, and St.-John's-wort. Herbs for Kids makes Minty Ginger herbal drops to soothe an upset stomach. The recommended dosages are on the bottle.

Other good options for stomach complaints are Friendly Flora/ Bifidus by Child Life and Rhino Tum-eez (wintergreen flavor) by Nutrition Now.

Homeopathic remedies can also effectively relieve children's abdominal pain. A product made by Standard Homeopathic Company called Nux Vomica and Carbo Veg combines two remedies in one tablet. If you can't find it, you can purchase the remedies individually and give one tablet of each. Another homeopathic formula good for stomachaches is

Gastrica by CompliMed. Homeopathic remedies good for intestinal gas include Ver by Deseret, Worms by CompliMed, and Gasalia by Boiron.

For chronic stomachaches, especially in a nervous child who becomes anxious over schoolwork, try Arsenicum alba 30x. Bach flower remedies can also help in cases with emotional causes. Rescue Remedy is one with universal application. For other natural options, see "Stomach-ache."

ABRASIONS, CUTS, SCRAPES, WOUNDS

CUTS AND scrapes are everyday occurrences for children, who experiment with everything from kitchen knives to broken glass, tend to run too fast, and often lose control in their exuberance to see and do.

 Home Care

SKINNED KNEES and other surface abrasions should be cleaned with a bath or plenty of warm water and a mild soap. Remove bits of dirt, sand, and asphalt, as these foreign objects may prevent healing and in some cases have even become incorporated into the healed skin like a tattoo. A thick, sterile, nonadherent dry dressing should be applied to protect the raw area from infection. The area needs rest so it will heal.

For deeper cuts, if the edges of the cut can be pulled together and held by bandaging, stitches need not be sought at the emergency room. Cuts on the head will heal in about three days, due to the ample blood supply there. Cuts on the body need to be held together for a week to make sure they are healed; ten days are required for cuts on the legs. A tetanus shot or booster is not needed for open cuts. Tetanus infection is thought to result only from a puncture wound that does not bleed, since bleeding pushes the infection out. Even for puncture wounds, the removal of dirt and any foreign substance followed by washing with soap and water is all that is normally required; but it is still a good idea to consult your pediatrician.

 Drug Treatment

While your pediatrician might advise a tetanus booster for something like a puncture wound due to a manure fork in the barnyard, the usual indoor cuts do not require pharmaceutical treatment. Over-the-counter antibiotic and cortisone ointments are available to ward off infection, but these drugs not only have side effects and other drawbacks but can actually worsen the injury. Many children are sensitive to them, and cortisone suppresses the immune system, which is the body's own weapon against infection. (See "Itching.")

 Natural Aids to Healing

Calendula ointment, made from the marigold flower, is a safe alternative treatment for cuts and scrapes. Calendula is also available in homeopathic form. Dramatic responses are often reported with this amazing ointment, which rapidly promotes healing of broken skin. Aloe vera gel is another popular topical option. After applying ointment, wrap the wound and leave it on for a few days. If new skin has not covered the wound, then apply new dressing.

Trauma and Traumeel ointments are good for a range of conditions from minor household accidents to major traumatic injuries. They contain homeopathic Hypericum, which stops nerve pain and takes the sting out; Arnica, which stops the body from overreacting to trauma; and Calendula, which promotes healing. The remedies also come as oral drops, which can be taken along with topical application at the rate of ten drops every fifteen minutes the first hour, then ten drops four times daily.

The recommended homeopathic remedy for a puncture wound is Ledum.

A poultice of bentonite clay (the powdered kind sold in health food stores for facials and skin treatments) can draw out infection.

For bruises and blunt trauma, see "Trauma."

Clay Saves Leg from Amputation

Author Ellen Brown lived for a while in Nicaragua, where her housekeeper had a nephew with a very badly infected leg. The boy was on antibiotics, but they were making him sick and the leg just kept getting worse. The doctor said that if the drugs did not work, the leg would have to be amputated. Mrs. Brown gave her housekeeper a five-pound bag of bentonite clay ($1.50 at the local Nicaraguan health food store) and told her how to make clay poultices with it. Two weeks later the housekeeper reported that, *"Gracias a Dios,"* the child's leg had healed. The doctor could not believe it and asked the mother what she had done. When she showed him the bag of clay, he remained baffled but said to keep it up, as it was working.

ABSCESSES (See Skin Infections)

ACCIDENT-PRONENESS (See Crawling)

ACNE

ACNE IS the most common skin disorder in the United States, afflicting more than sixteen million American teenagers. Pimples result when sebaceous glands at the base of hair follicles get clogged with oil, causing inflammation and attracting bacteria. Bacteria can turn blackheads and whiteheads into red, inflamed pimples. White blood cells rush to the area, causing swelling as they fight the infection. Changing hormones can aggravate the condition, leaving teenagers particularly susceptible. Other aggravating factors include stress, poor diet, and food allergies. Milk products are common suspects. Blemish problems have also been traced to certain drugs (including over-the-counter drugs like aspirin)[6] and to a reaction to the fluoride in city water.[7]

Cystic acne is a serious form of the disease that can result in permanent pits and scars. The tendency to develop cystic acne or to have oily skin may be hereditary.

 Drug Treatment

A WIDE range of drugs is used on this ubiquitous condition, including antibiotics, retinoids, birth-control pills, and over-the-counter creams and gels. Their drawbacks range from ineffectiveness to serious health hazards.

Antibiotics have been a mainstay of treatment, even for mild outbreaks of acne. The theory was that antibiotics reduce the chance of secondary infection in plugged oil glands and preclude scarring. But if the drugs ever had this effect, they no longer seem to be working well. Several recent studies have shown that acne-causing bacteria have developed strains that are resistant to both oral and topical antibiotics.[8]

Accutane (isotretinoin) is one of a class of vitamin-A derivatives called retinoids. Accutane can produce dramatic clearing of lesions in severe, recalcitrant cystic acne that is unresponsive to conventional therapy.[9] Unfortunately, the usefulness of this "wonder drug" is severely limited by its major risks of side effects and birth defects. Nearly everyone receiving therapeutic doses of Accutane experiences drying and inflammation of the lips and chapping, itching, inflammation, and dryness of the skin. Some patients experience dryness in the eyes and an increased sensitivity to sunlight, symptoms that may not go away after the drug course is completed. Some patients also suffer vague aches and pains in the muscles and bones. Some lose a portion of their hair.[10] Specialists now recommend that Accutane be used only on patients with deep-seated cystic or pustular acne that is unresponsive to any other form of treatment, who have been carefully screened for contraindications by physicians thoroughly familiar with the drug.[11] Mild acne may be treated with the topical cream Retin-A (tretinoin), a milder retinoid subject to side effects similar to Accutane's but in lighter form. **Caution: Retinoids are likely to cause sun sensitivity. Their prescription should always come with warnings to use sunscreens.**

The birth-control pill is thought to ameliorate acne because estrogen suppresses the sebaceous glands' production of oil.[12] The Pill has been used as an acne treatment since the sixties, when it contained quite high levels of estrogen. When doses were later lowered to safer levels, however, improvements in the complexions of Pill-takers became much less common, and many women noticed a worsening of acne when they stopped taking the drug. Side effects of the Pill can even include acne.[13]

Over-the-counter topical acne remedies have also proliferated, including a variety of creams and gels based on drying agents like benzoyl peroxide; but the products remain only marginally effective and are quite drying to the skin. They take four to six weeks to work if they work at all, and when they are discontinued the acne comes back. While rubbing with alcohol tends to cut grease and dry the skin, some dermatologists feel that this drying effect actually stimulates the manufacture of oil. Medicated cleansers are generally a waste of money, since the medication washes off. Granular facial scrubs work no better than a washcloth, and facial saunas can actually aggravate acne.

 Tracking the Cause

HOMEOPATHIC DOCTORS view the skin as an important organ of elimination. If its eruptions are suppressed, toxins that the skin is trying to eliminate will be driven farther into the body, manifesting later as more serious chronic disease. Suppression with drugs must be done continually, since when they are discontinued the problem comes right back. A lasting cure for acne needs to address the cause. Likely causes include dietary offenders, environmental toxins, and certain drugs.

To find out if food allergies are the problem, acne sufferers can try going on an elimination diet, then systematically adding suspect foods back in.[14] If a food is definitely implicated by the return of symptoms, eliminate it from the diet for at least three months, then try it cautiously. If no reaction occurs, eat it in moderation.

Teenagers in underdeveloped countries whose diets are based on vegetables and grains are substantially less prone to complexion problems than Americans. For people willing to undergo a radical dietary overhaul, macrobiotic fare (whole grains, no milk, few or no animal products) has been reported to work miracles on blemishes.[15] There is no scientific proof that chocolate, nuts, or sodas trigger outbreaks, but anecdotal evidence suggests that they do, and Chinese medicine has an explanation: These foods congest the liver, preventing it from clearing toxins, which are eliminated instead through the pores of the skin. Since these foods have no redeeming dietary virtues, cutting them out can't hurt. Eating less fat and more fruits and vegetables can also make your skin less oily. Fresh-squeezed fruit and vegetable juices—particularly carrot and cucumber—help oxygenate the blood and the skin it feeds.

Acne around the mouth can indicate digestive problems. Digestive enzymes can help in these cases, along with general nutritional support.

If acne can be traced to drugs or environmental toxins, try to eliminate those triggers.

 ## Natural Acne Relief

THE BODY'S elimination of underlying toxins can also be stimulated by herbal and homeopathic remedies, which can resolve the problem for good.

Margarite Acne Pills are a very effective Chinese patent remedy that works on this toxin-eliminating principle. Chinese doctors believe that toxins build up in the blood and come out through the skin.

A gemmotherapy that helps clear acne is Oriental Plane Tree by Dolisos.

Effective homeopathic acne products currently on the market include Clear-AC by Hyland's (which comes both as an oral tablet and a topical cream), Bacticin by CompliMed, and Nelson Acne Gel.

Herpacine, a formula by Dr. Wayne Diamond, is a total skin-support system that is high in antioxidants. It works from the inside out to clear acne and improve the quality of the skin.

Colostrum (the first mammary secretions of lactating cows) can help reduce infection. It is now available in pill form.

Recurring Acne Cleared

Nineteen-year-old Kelley was quite self-conscious about her complexion, which was severely stricken with acne. She began taking Margarite Acne Pills, and in two weeks, her complexion began to clear. In three weeks, it looked great.

Home Skin Treatments, Cleansing, and Tonics

SOME SIMPLE home skin-care measures can also help keep symptoms under control:

1. Wash with ordinary soap and water. Dr. Bronner's pure castile soap is good. Once or twice a day is sufficient, since washing your skin too much can actually worsen acne.

2. Resist the urge to pick at blemishes, a habit that increases the risk of pits and scars.

3. Use either no cosmetics or the water-based kind. Avoid greasy hair dressings. Wear your hair away from your face.

4. For a facial scrub, try oatmeal. Make a paste of rolled oats and water, let it dry on your face, then wash it off.

5. If you feel you need a commercial product, use natural formulations such as aloe, which can give quick skin relief.

6. If you can, spend a week at the beach. Sunshine brings oil to the surface of the skin, while saltwater acts as an astringent and cleans out the skin. (Prescription drug users should consult a pharmacist before sunbathing. For other precautions, see "Sunburn.")

7. To draw oil out, try applying healing clay or a paste of baking soda and water to blemishes. Bentonite clay for facials is available at health food stores. Other possibilities are a dab of toothpaste or tea tree oil.[16]

Cystic Acne Cleared with Bentonite

A young man who worked in the sun and sweated a great deal had cystic acne all over his back. He was advised to brush his skin with a natural-bristle brush before showering, then apply bentonite clay to his back every night. The remedy drew the toxins from his acne and cleared it up.

ADD, ADHD (See Attention Deficit Hyperactivity Disorder)

AGGRESSIVENESS (See Anger)

ALLERGIES, HAY FEVER

ALLERGIES ARE responsible for one in five visits to the pediatrician and are the leading reason for hospitalization in children. By far the most common allergy is hay fever, or allergic rhinitis—an inflammation of the nasal passages caused by an irritant—which strikes some six million children annually.

An increased incidence of allergies in industrialized countries has been linked to an increase in pollutants, chemicals, pesticides, and other allergy-provoking foreign substances. Several studies reported in 1997 also linked allergies and diabetes (both autoimmune diseases) to immunization and a decreased incidence of childhood infections. The suggested explanation is that the evolving immune system needs to keep busy. If it has no invaders to cope with, it turns its defenses on otherwise harmless stimuli. In one study, nearly three hundred children in Guinea-Bissau were tested for allergic reactions to airborne allergens. Allergies (asthma, eczema, hay fever, etc.) were found to be significantly more common in children who had never had measles. Exposure to hepatitis A and tuberculosis has also been shown to afford immunity to allergies. In two recent studies conducted in Italy, allergies were found to be less common among the poor and among people who grew up in big families or unsanitary surroundings.[17] It seems that exposure of the young immune system to germs may be necessary to its proper development.

 Drug Treatment

THE ANTIHISTAMINES familiar in treating colds are actually more helpful in treating allergies, since allergies result from the *inappropriate* release of histamine into the bloodstream. Antihistamines have been available since the 1940s. A drawback of the older versions (Benadryl, Allerest, Chlor-Trimeton) is that they produce drowsiness. A later-model antihistamine called Seldane (terfenadine) overcame this defect, but the FDA withdrew it from the market in 1997 when a rash of deaths was attributed to its use in conjunction with certain other drugs. Other drugs of this type (Claritin, Zyrtec, Allegra) are still on the market, but the chemical structures and modes of action of these drugs are all similar to Seldane's, making them all suspect.[18]

Steroid-containing nasal sprays are also available now for the treatment of hay fever (Vancenase, Flonase). The sprays are thought to reduce the serious systemic effects of steroids taken by mouth, since they hit only the nose rather than the whole body; but their safety still remains to be established. The new steroid inhalers for asthma, which were also thought to be safer than steroids taken by mouth, have now been found to have some of the same side effects as oral steroids. (See "Asthma.") Other drawbacks of the sprays are that they take two to four days to work and can irritate the nose. The hazards of steroids in general are discussed in the introduction.

Caution: For the treatment of hay fever, decongestants or decongestant/antihistamine combinations should be avoided, since they can cause a rebound effect and are potentially addictive if used for more than a few days. They are particularly hazardous when used for hay fever, since it tends to last more than a few days.

Allergy Shots

ALLERGY DESENSITIZATION injections are generally reserved for people with severe allergies, since they are a long and expensive commitment with an uncertain outcome. A typical course can take three to five years, and it may be a full year before any improvement is seen. The required once- or twice-weekly office visits have been called annuities for allergists. Whether the shots actually reduce or eliminate allergies remains to be established, since many young people outgrow their allergies even without treatment. A study reported in *The New England Journal of Medicine* in January 1997 found that most children with asthma don't benefit from allergy shots.[19]

Natural Remedies

ALTHOUGH A tendency to develop allergies is often hereditary, the allergies may not become manifest if the adrenal glands are producing enough cortisol. Nutritional supplements can aid this process, including vitamin C and pantothenic acid.

Effective homeopathic remedies are available that help desensitize the body to specific allergens. A number of companies, including Deseret, Molecular Biologicals, and CompliMed, make good combination homeopathic remedies identified by allergen. Combination homeopathic remedies are also available for people who don't know what they are allergic to, including Allerdrain and Aller-Total by Futureplex.

A gemmotherapy that can help relieve allergies is Black Currant by Dolisos.

For congestion, try hot tea made with natural decongestants such as fenugreek, anise, and sage. Garlic, onions, and hot and spicy foods can also thin out mucus.

Exercise is a natural adrenaline stimulant that causes the bronchioles to dilate and helps relieve allergic attacks.[20]

F. Batmanghelidj, M.D., in *Your Body's Many Cries for Water,* asserts that asthma and allergies are diseases of water dehydration. He has seen many cases cured simply by increasing the patient's intake of pure water.[21] For protocol, see "Nutrition."

For other suggestions, see "Asthma."

 Avoiding the Cause

AN OBVIOUS precaution is to reduce the exposure of allergic children to known allergens like cats or down pillows. For allergies to airborne substances, an air conditioner or air filter in your heating system can help. So can a humidifier or vaporizer, but it can also aggravate some allergies by producing a moist environment that encourages the growth of allergy-producing molds.

Food allergies account for many less obvious childhood symptoms, including eczema (skin rash), chronic coughs and bronchitis, diarrhea, migraine headaches, colitis, and even otitis media.[22] Again, substantial improvement may result from avoiding the common offenders—eggs, milk, nuts, soy, wheat, and the nightshades (tomatoes, potatoes, green peppers, eggplant). If you suspect your child has a food allergy, try eliminating these foods, then adding them back into the diet one by one. If a food is definitely implicated by the return of symptoms, eliminate it from the diet for at least three months, then try it cautiously. If no reaction occurs, it can be eaten by the child in moderation.[23] This process can require substantial effort by the parent, but it is worth the trouble, since children often outgrow their allergies. If the food isn't avoided, the allergy is more likely to remain.[24] For substitutes for allergy-provoking foods, see "Nutrition."

Desensitization can be started even before the child is born. If one parent has allergies, the chances are one in three that the child will, too; and if both parents have them, the chances are two in three. Mothers who suspect food allergies can start by passing up allergy-causing foods while they're pregnant and nursing. Eggs, milk products, nuts, and peanut butter are leading suspects to avoid.[25]

An unsuspected cause of allergies may be parasites. See "Parasites."

ANAL FISSURE

AN ANAL fissure is a crack or break in the lining of the mucosa at the anal opening, typically resulting from the passage of a large, hard, dry bowel movement. If anal fissures are associated with cracks around the mouth, the underlying cause is usually sensitivity to some food.

 Natural Home Remedies

CALENDULA CREAM applied after each bowel movement helps promote healing. Meanwhile, likely foods should be systematically eliminated from the diet. Common offenders include citrus, tomatoes, nuts, dairy products, soy products, and corn, but there are many other possibilities.

ANAL RING (See Colic)

ANEMIA

ANEMIA IS a condition in which body tissues get insufficient oxygen, either because there aren't enough red blood cells in circulation or because the blood is low in hemoglobin, an essential protein. Anemia can result from blood loss or from the destruction of blood cells or their insufficient production in the body.

Childhood anemias include hemolytic anemia and iron-deficiency anemia. Hemolytic anemia is a blood disorder in which red blood cells are destroyed at an unusually high rate. It is usually hereditary, although it can also be caused by drugs or certain types of infections. Treatment needs to be prescribed by a physician. The most common cause of anemia in children, however, is iron deficiency, usually due to a lack of absorbable iron in the diet. Iron is a necessary constituent of hemoglobin. Anemia may also result from a lack of other nutrients, including folic acid and vitamin B_{12}.

Menstruating teenage girls, teens on fad diets lacking in iron, children under three who drink large amounts of milk to the exclusion of other animal proteins, and premature babies are all particularly prone to iron-deficiency anemia. The condition is common in infants who have been drinking only cow's milk for their first several months of life. Human babies do not become anemic if breast-fed, since they are able to absorb the iron from human breast milk; but the iron in cow's milk is species-specific for calves. Cow's milk is difficult to absorb and can cause intestinal bleeding in babies. The safest approach is to refrain from giving it until after the baby is one year old. After eight months of age, the bottle-fed baby is usually started on solid foods, which will provide some iron.

Other types of anemia (for example, sickle cell anemia) are hereditary. Anemia may also result from the use of drugs, from infestations of parasites such as hookworm and tapeworm, and from malaria. A serious case could indicate leukemia.

Conventional Treatment

IRON-DEFICIENCY ANEMIA is usually treated with supplemental iron, but iron supplements aren't very effective in rebuilding the blood, can be constipating, and are highly toxic in overdose. They also take a long time to be absorbed; several weeks are required before blood iron reaches optimum levels. Enteric-coated supplements can't be effectively absorbed and should be avoided.

Anemia may also be treated with supplements of folic acid or other nutrients in which the patient's blood levels are low. Serious types of anemia caused by bleeding of the digestive tract are conventionally corrected by surgery.

 Natural Remedies

NO IRON supplements should be used unless definitely needed, but if they are needed, ferrous gluconate is an absorbable form. A good option is liquid Floradix, an iron-containing herbal combination that is easily absorbed.

Chlorophyll, the blood of plants, has a chemical composition very similar to hemoglobin and can help rebuild the blood. It is particularly abundant in green vegetables; however, eating enough green vegetables to reverse anemia is difficult, particularly for kids. The easier alternative is supplemental chlorophyll (two ounces in water two to three times daily) or "green" pills: spirulina, chlorella, or Ultimate Green by Nature's Secret. Hemaplex by Nature's Plus is also good, but it comes as a large capsule that only older children are able to swallow. The dose is one daily.

A gemmotherapy that can help relieve anemia is Tamarisk by Dolisos.

The homeopathic treatment for anemia is Ferrum phos taken as a cell salt in a 6x potency three to four times daily. It tastes like candy, melts as soon as it touches the tongue, and doesn't cause constipation like most iron supplements. It will build the blood over a period of several months. It also helps the immune system of the child with chronic colds, and it is a good remedy for bleeding problems, including chronic nosebleeds and long, heavy periods.

ANGER, TEMPER TANTRUMS, BREATH-HOLDING, AGGRESSIVENESS

A *TEMPER tantrum* is a form of communication by which the verbally inadequate fifteen- to eighteen-month-old child expresses anger and frustration. Almost all children pass through this phase. Boys seem more prone to tantrums, perhaps because their speech development tends to be slower than girls'. If the tantrums continue beyond eighteen months, other factors should be considered, including a poor diet, heavy-metal poisoning, worms, and anemia.

Breath-holding is sometimes seen in babies of around fifteen months, an age when they are attempting to establish some autonomy and independence. They want to play with dangerous things, eat nonfoods, and explore the environment. Their parents say "No!" The response is to cry angrily and hold the breath, sometimes to the point of turning blue or even passing out. This can be quite worrisome to parents, but the child actually suffers no harm unless he or she has a real breathing problem, since the body starts breathing on its own once the child gets dizzy or blacks out momentarily. You should check with your pediatrician, however, for breathing defects.

By the time a child is six years old, he should be able to express or sublimate his anger without acting it out; but despite the best domestic care, some children seem to stray from society's rules. *Aggressiveness* includes actions like arson, delinquency, and general disobedience. Psychotherapy may help, but nutritional and environmental factors should also be considered, including heavy-metal toxicity, hypoglycemia, and food sensitivity. A hair analysis and other tests from an appropriate professional can give clues. See "Heavy-metal Poisoning," "Allergies," "Hypoglycemia."

 ## Behavioral Approaches

UNDER THE "time out" approach to temper tantrums and breath-holding, the parent doesn't reward the behavior with attention, either positive (cuddling and love) or negative (spankings and punishment). The parent simply turns her back on the child and walks into the next room, closing the door; or sends the child to his room and closes the door. There is some question, however, whether we haven't gone too far in avoiding spankings. In countries where physical discipline is condoned, children seem better behaved. Only a couple of spankings, delivered when bad bahavior first manifests, are generally sufficient to make the point. But the authors themselves are split on this issue, on which whole books have been written.

Meanwhile, parents should check the emotions they are projecting onto the child. A child who is angry enough to hold his breath to the point of turning blue may be responding to an angry tone from parents. "No" can be said in a loving way.

 ## Natural Remedies

RESCUE REMEDY—a Bach flower remedy—put in a spray bottle and sprayed about the room works remarkably well to calm children who are angry, agitated, or upset.

Chamomilla 30x or 30c is a homeopathic remedy that helps calm cranky, irritable children and quell temper tantrums. For the child who is shrieking, defiant, and constipated, try Cina 30x.

Ignatia 30c is the appropriate homeopathic remedy to relieve an urge to engage in breath-holding. Give the child three pellets three times a day for twenty days a month over a period of several months.

For other remedies for bad moods and temperamental behavior, see "Attention Deficit Hyperactivity Disorder," "Depression," and "Anxiety."

ANIMAL BITES, RABIES

ANIMAL BITES are common in children, who tend to be careless when approaching cats and dogs. Bites should be cleansed carefully with soap and clean water. (See "Abrasions.") Some need suturing, but animal bites typically do not get infected, and a tetanus booster is usually not required. Your doctor will decide.

Rabies is a serious viral infection caused by the bite of an infected animal. It is usually fatal unless the bitten person receives a hyperimmune serum, but parents need not get unduly alarmed if their children get bitten, because rabies is very rare and the possibility that someone's pet has it is highly unlikely. Carriers include dogs and cats, as well as skunks, bats, and other wild animals. Dogs who have bitten humans who have not recently been vaccinated must be quarantined. If the animal dies, an autopsy is done to find evidence of the disease.

See also "Cat Scratch Disease."

ANKLE, SPRAINED (See Sprains)

ANOREXIA, ANOREXIA NERVOSA, BULIMIA

ANOREXIA, OR loss of appetite, can accompany the flu, a stomachache, a bladder infection, a sore throat, or other common ills. An unsuspected cause in babies may be the ingestion of too much cow's milk, leading to iron-deficiency anemia. (See "Anemia.")

Anorexia nervosa is an eating disorder that is considered a psychological problem. It is usually seen in adolescent girls who feel insecure, particularly about their appearance. A loved one may have said something like "If you could just lose a few pounds . . ." This insecurity sets off a cycle of not eating, losing weight, and visits to the psychiatrist.

Bulimia nervosa is an eating disorder generally found in teenage girls and young women, characterized by episodes of eating large quantities of food in a short time, followed by severe food restriction and often vomiting, laxative abuse, or excessive exercising to prevent weight gain. Health risks include major disturbance of the blood chemistry and rupture of the stomach, which, in the extreme case, can cause sudden death. More common adverse effects are zinc deficiency and harm to the teeth: Stomach acid constantly washing over the teeth dissolves the enamel, causing lasting damage. If the illness is severe, the sufferer may also fail to make normal relationships and become withdrawn, moody, and intolerant. As with all eating disorders, the greatest risks are from suicide or self-harm as a result of emotional disturbances.[26]

 Natural Remedies

IF ANOREXIA is due to anemia, an iron tonic can help boost the appetite for solids. Floradix is a good brand available in health food stores.

For anorexia nervosa, zinc therapy may help. After a few weeks of not eating, mineral deficiencies become the compelling reason for rejecting food. Without an optimum level of zinc in the body, food has no taste or tastes quite bad. A taste test with a zinc solution will reveal this deficiency. The anorexic person notes no disagreeable taste, while a normal person with sufficient zinc in the tissues will spit out the solution immediately.

Platina is a homeopathic remedy that can help in cases in which a girl believes she is overweight when others feel her weight is normal.

A gemmotherapy called Lime Tree by Dolisos can help in cases of both anorexia and bulimia.

For remedies for the anxiety underlying eating disorders, see "Anxiety."

ANUS, ITCHY (See Itching, Anal)

ANXIETY, PHOBIAS

ANXIETY IS a feeling of worry accompanied by physical symptoms: palpitation, pain, constriction in the chest, a lump in the throat. Arguments or tensions at home or school, worry about exams or social life, even frightening or violent movies can trigger it in children. Anxiety is a normal reaction to stress, which causes a release of adrenaline into the system. Adrenaline alerts the heart, the sweat glands, the vision, and the muscles, getting the body ready for fight or flight. The result can be not only psychological symptoms (tension, fear, difficulty concentrating, apprehension) but physical symptoms including tachycardia (rapid heartbeat), increased blood pressure, hyperventilation, palpitations (irregular or strong heartbeats), tremors, headache, and sweating. Less obvious effects may include weakened immunity, nervousness, indigestion, problems concentrating, sleeplessness, and chronic fatigue.

Abnormal anxiety is an adrenaline rush without an obvious cause. Phobias are another form of anxiety disorder—claustrophobia, agoraphobia (fear of going out or leaving home), acrophobia (fear of heights). Fear of the dark and fear of going to school are common phobias of children. Other anxiety disorders include obsessions (obsessive-compulsive disorder, compulsive handwashing, counting rituals), panic attacks, hair pulling, nail biting, hypochondria, Tourette's syndrome, and eating disorders. (See "Anorexia.")

 Conventional Treatment

PROZAC AND its corollaries (Zoloft, Paxil, Wellbutrin, Luvox) are the current drug favorites for anxiety, depression, and a host of other ills. Although not labeled for pediatric use, these popular drugs are now being prescribed even for young children. Zoloft has been approved to treat obsessive-compulsive disorder in children six and older, and Luvox is approved for children eight and older; but both drugs are being used in younger children. A late addition to the depression/anxiety pharmacopia is a drug called Effexor, which is also being prescribed for children and young adults.

These drugs obliterate anxiety and depression by numbing the whole system. Common side effects include disruption of sleep patterns, nervousness, nausea and (ironically) anxiety. A more alarming side effect is outbursts of violence. Some 3.5 percent of patients who weren't suicidal before treatment with Prozac get that way on the drug, and it has been blamed for homicides, generating a spate of lawsuits.[27] The concern is that psychotropic drugs unbalance brain chemicals. Eric Harris, one of the Colorado school shooting perpetrators, had been taking Luvox. Kip Kinkel, the Oregon school shooter, had been on Prozac.

Caution: If prescription antianxiety or insomnia drugs are already being used, discontinue or switch remedies only under professional supervision.

Tracking the Cause

BETTER THAN suppressing symptoms with drugs is to find the cause of anxiety and assist the child in eliminating it. Dietary stressors should be considered, and counseling may help, but children and especially teenagers want sympathy, understanding, and support more than advice. The function of the teenage years is to develop character traits for adult life. Dependence on either drugs or parental or professional oversight defeats this process. Character development in teenagers is remarkably rapid. The class "nerd" of eighth grade may be the student-body president of twelfth grade. One of the joys of parenthood is to watch this flowering of character traits, something that occurs of its own accord in children and young adults left to work out their own problems. Support them, encourage them, and watch them grow.

Watching Them Flower

After a move from a friendly school in Nairobi, Kenya, to an unfriendly school in Honduras, the daughter of one of the authors became seriously depressed and uncommunicative and suffered from nightmares and anxiety attacks. Her parents feared the move had scarred their daughter for life; but in fact, having few friends in Honduras motivated her to devote all her time to her studies. She had gotten mediocre grades in Kenya but became first in her class in Honduras. She graduated valedictorian and class president from her high school in Guatemala, where she formed many enduring friendships. She went on to become a Presidential Scholar, earning an award from President Bill Clinton.

Natural Alternatives

WHILE YOU are waiting for your child to achieve insight and resolution, there are safe and effective natural remedies for assuaging the attacks of adrenaline that come with worry and anxiety.

Rescue Remedy is a Bach flower remedy that is excellent for the child who is anxious over a move, separation from parents, or the first day of school. Cherry Plum is another Bach flower remedy good for anxiety.

Aromatherapy is calming and relaxing. Chamomile oil is good for the child who has trouble relaxing or is hyperactive, nervous, or upset. Lavender oil is also calming: Put it in the bedroom, near or on the child's pillow or on a rag placed near the bed, or burn a lavender-scented candle in the room. Some pillows are made with lavender seeds in them.

Herbs that are safe and effective for treating anxiety in children include skullcap, oats, valerian, and St.-John's-wort. Research shows that herbs can be as effective as prescription drugs for calming the nerves, without their dangerous side effects.[28] Eclectic Institute makes Skullcap Oats in a sweet glycerin base that tastes good to children. Herbs for Kids makes a combination herbal formula for nervous and anxious children called Valerian Super Calm, along with a product called Valerian Certified Organic Drops. Chamomile Calm by Herbs for Kids is a combination of chamomile and skullcap in an alcohol-free formula that helps calm crying, irritable children. Herbs for Kids makes a St.-John's-wort product specifically for children.

Even safer than herbs are homeopathic remedies for alleviating childhood anxieties. Categorized by type of anxiety, they include:

> For dread of the future: Argentum nitricum
> For a letdown or sad event: Ignatia
> For anxiety from hot weather: Pulsatilla
> For anxiety from the aftereffects of a fright (for example, a car accident): Aconite
> For anxiety that is worse when alone: Arsenicum

For anxiety that is worse at nightfall: Phosphorus

For anticipatory anxiety (nervousness before a speech or an exam): Gelsenium 30x (three tablets as needed, up to four times a day).

For phobias and to bring out and eliminate the underlying cause of anxieties, constitutional homeopathic treatment from a qualified practitioner is often effective. Children respond extremely well to homeopathic treatment, which can change their lives.

For obsessive-compulsive disorder (an anxiety disorder that can manifest in obsessively counting things and other abnormal ritual behavior), a gemmotherapy called Lime Tree by Dolisos can help.

In some circumstances, simple relaxation can be as effective as drugs in alleviating anxiety. In a study of patients about to undergo surgery, acupressure (a form of massage) and relaxation/meditation tapes were found to work as well as or better than Valium.[29] Music therapy and color therapy are other possibilities. Blue light is calming.

Anxiety attacks may be triggered not only by stress and external fears but by hypoglycemia or food allergies. The consumption of some sensitizing food or a dose of sugar can make the blood sugar rise, then plummet. When the blood sugar falls, the body assumes it is under attack and releases adrenaline. This may explain a child's frightening dream at two A.M. after being given a dish of ice cream to get him into bed at a reasonable hour (ice cream is 20 percent sugar). (See "Night Terrors.") Stimulants such as caffeine (found in coffee, tea, colas, and other soft drinks), *ma huang* (herba ephedra, or ephedrine, found in over-the-counter diet aids and in Herbal Ecstasy), alcohol (found in some cough medicines), and chocolate can also induce symptoms of anxiety.

See also "Stress," "Insomnia," "Stage Fright."

APPENDICITIS

APPENDICITIS IS a bacterial inflammation of the appendix, an append-age usually found at the cecum lying at the lower right side of the abdomen. It typically results when something like an apple seed or nut gets caught in the appendix, which then gets infected. Symptoms start with discomfort around the navel. In an hour or so, the pain migrates to the lower right side of the abdomen. Sufferers say it feels like the worst attack of gas they ever had, but the pain does not disappear after a bowel movement. Another distinguishing feature of appendicitis is that the muscles of the abdomen are usually rigid over the lower right side. When these symptoms are present, a consultation with a surgeon and possibly a white blood count are advised. Because appendicitis is a bacterial problem, the white count is usually elevated to at least twelve thousand. Under those circumstances, the patient is normally taken to surgery within the hour to avoid the possibility that the appendix will rupture and spread infection to the abdominal cavity, causing peritoni-tis, which can be fatal.

Appendicitis may run in families, particularly families with a tendency toward constipation, since hard feces lodged in the appendix can lead to obstruction and infection. However, this problem may be due to family dietary habits rather than genetics. See "Constipation."

For chronic (as opposed to acute) appendicitis, homeopathic remedies may be tried as an alternative to surgery. Consult a homeopath.

Symptoms Mimicking Appendicitis

Symptoms apparently indicating appendicitis may have other causes. A fourteen-year-old patient had all of the indications of appendicitis, including an elevated white blood count. The surgeon opened the abdomen and found, to his embarrassment, that it was normal. Three weeks after the patient returned home, the symptoms recurred. Questioning revealed no changes in his lifestyle other than beginning an antibiotic for acne. When he stopped the antibiotic, the pain disappeared. Apparently, the drug had affected his intestinal function.

APPETITE, LOSS OF (See Anorexia)

APHTHOUS ULCERS (See Canker Sores)

ARTHRITIS, CHILDHOOD

ARTHRITIS, OR inflammation of the joints, is unusual in children. The most common form is *traumatic arthritis,* which results from some injury. The joint has been hit or twisted, causing fluid to fill it and press on the nerves, making it hot, swollen, and tender. More serious is *juvenile rheumatoid arthritis,* an inflammation that seems to follow an infection, most likely strep. It can cause stiff joints and pain that becomes chronic. A form of childhood arthritis is also associated with acute rheumatic fever, but it goes away when the disease does.

 Conventional Treatment

CONVENTIONAL TREATMENT for juvenile rheumatoid arthritis includes prophylactic antibiotic therapy or cortisone drugs. Unfortunately, these drugs can have quite serious side effects when taken for long periods. (See Introduction.) For other forms of juvenile joint pain, analgesic (painkilling) drugs are used.

Nondrug Treatment

FOR TEMPORARY joint pain in children, the conservative approach is rest, ice packs for twenty-four hours, then heat.

For juvenile rheumatoid arthritis, homeopaths maintain that conventional drug treatment with cortisone merely drives the infection deeper into the body and worsens the condition. To bring the infection out and eliminate it, a remedy called Staph/Strep, made by the German homeopathic company Staufen, is quite effective. Comparable series therapy is available in the United States from Deseret.

Pancreatic enzymes have also been shown to help. In 1996 Russian researchers found that a German enzyme formulation called Wobenzym significantly reduced the number of actively inflamed joints in children with juvenile rheumatoid arthritis.[30] Wobenzym tablets are manufactured by MUCOS Pharma GmbH and are available by mail-order from Naturally Vitamins in Scottsdale, Arizona, telephone 800-899-4499. They should be taken on an empty stomach not less than forty-five minutes before, or two hours after, meals.

ASPARTAME (ARTIFICIAL SWEETENER) ADDICTION

ASPARTAME (NUTRASWEET and other brands) is an artificial sweetener that is about 160 times as sweet as sugar. It is now found in about four thousand foods and many soft drinks. Added for the purpose of reducing caloric intake while satisfying the sweet tooth of those who want to lose weight, it is consumed by millions of people, many of them children. Although aspartame is labeled as a food and considered safe, the FDA gets more calls about its adverse effects than any other "food." Reported side effects include blindness, eye pain, tinnitus, intolerance to noise, decreased hearing, seizures, headaches, dizziness, confusion, memory loss, sleepiness, numbness in limbs, slurring of speech, tremors, depression, irritability, anxiety, nausea, diarrhea, hives, weight gain, aggravated low blood sugar, and chronic fatigue.[31]

Worse, research now shows that aspartame consumption can actually *increase* the appetite and cause weight *gain*. When the taste buds detect sweet material, they send a message to the thalamus in the brain: "Incoming sugar!" The thalamus then sends a message to the pancreas, which activates beta cells to put insulin into the bloodstream to metabolize the anticipated sugar onslaught and store it in the cells. But there is no sugar onslaught, so the sugar already in the bloodstream is stored instead. The blood sugar then falls, and appetite for more energy-producing sugar increases. Many people have other symptoms besides an increased appetite when the blood sugar falls, including headaches, migraine, anxiety, weakness, somnolence, hyperactivity, seizures, and depression.

The insulin imbalance created by habitual aspartame ingestion is also thought by some researchers to precipitate insulin resistance, a common feature of diabetes. When sugar is eaten, the body produces insulin to burn it as energy. If there is too much insulin, the cells become desensitized to it. Following aspartame ingestion, insulin is sent in but not actually used, so the excess insulin attacks the cells, which no longer respond normally. This effect is called insulin resistance.

The solution is to avoid artificially sweetened foods and drinks. But that doesn't mean replacing artificially sweetened soft drinks with sugared soft drinks, which are high in both sugar and phosphoric acid, pulling calcium from the bones. For healthy alternatives, see "Nutrition."

ASTHMA

ASTHMA IS the most common chronic childhood disease and is increasing in incidence by up to 50 percent every ten years.[32] The condition now afflicts one in four children in industrialized countries, including an estimated 4.8 million American children. A breathing disorder characterized by wheezing, difficulty exhaling, and often coughing, asthma is caused by a constriction of the tiny muscles in the bronchial tubes that makes expiration difficult. It is usually due to some allergy, sensitivity, or air pollutant that irritates the lining of the bronchi. Once considered nonfatal, asthma now kills thousands of children annually and is responsible for more admissions to the hospital than any other childhood condition.[33]

Asthma has come to be regarded not so much as a disease as a disturbed breathing pattern. The breathing pattern changes in response to some emotional or environmental stress.[34] Foods can trigger the disturbance—dairy products, red meat, chocolate, refined sugar, MSG (monosodium glutamate). Other potential triggers include exercise, cold weather, and environmental irritants like dust mites, mold, animal dander, and chemical odors. The high level of airborne pollutants in industrialized countries is a leading suspect in the growing incidence of asthma. Cockroaches are a major trigger in inner-city children. And a cluster of infant deaths from lung disease has been linked to a toxic fungus found in the home.[35]

A Scottish study reported in the medical journal *Thorax* on August 22, 2000, found that diets rich in junk food could also be culprits behind the rapid rise in childhood asthma and allergies. A direct relationship was found between the frequency of eating at fast-food outlets and the incidence of asthma. A comparison of children with and without asthma symptoms showed that those with the lowest intakes of vegetables, milk, vitamin E, and minerals were more likely to suffer from the disease, without regard to other factors like family size, affluence, and parental smoking.[36]

Antibiotics and early childhood immunizations are also suspected of contributing to asthma incidence.[37] (See "Allergies.") Children who have repeated respiratory infections, subjecting them to repeated courses of antibiotics, are more likely to develop asthma.[38] Childhood asthma can also develop in babies given cortisone for a skin rash or as a reaction to aspirin.

 Drug Treatment

IRONICALLY THE drugs used to treat asthma are other suspects underlying the surge in deaths from the disease. Aerosol preparations in metered-dose inhalers for dilating the bronchial tubes afford a false sense of security in the face of a dangerous condition, while drug side effects compound the problem. All antiasthma medications can produce life-threatening reactions, and the likelihood of these reactions is multiplied by the increased use of the medications.[39]

Two types of asthma drugs are common today: controller (long-term) drugs and rescue (quick-relief) drugs.[40] Controller drugs suppress the underlying inflammation associated with asthma, thus preventing or reducing the risk of an asthma attack. They aren't effective if reserved for acute attacks; they must be used regularly. They include steroid inhalers (beclomethasone, triamcinolone, flunisolide, fluticasone, budesonide), oral steroids (methylprednisone, prednisone, and prednisolone in pill form), cromolyn, nedocromil, leukotriene modifiers (Singulare and others), and long-acting bronchodilators (salmeterol, sustained-release albuterol, and theophylline). Rescue drugs do not treat the underlying inflammation but are used to alleviate the symptoms of asthma flare-ups or acute asthma attacks. They include short-acting beta2-agonists (albuterol, bitolterol, pirbuterol), anticholinergics, and oral steroids.

Steroids reduce inflammation, opening the airways of the chest, and they suppress much of the immune system's response to allergens. However, the drugs don't cure the problem. They act mainly by inhibiting the body's reaction to it. The downside is that when extra steroids are taken, the adrenals quit making their own; so when natural steroids are needed to cope with stressful emergencies, they're no longer available. Side effects include emotional and growth problems in children, as well as bone loss, weight gain, easy bruising, and cataracts. These drugs should be used only short-term and after all other treatments fail. In children, they cannot be used for asthma attacks more than about four times a year without significant adverse effects.

Caution: If your child has a serious asthmatic condition, it is particularly important that he or she be under the regular care of a physician specializing in the field. Asthma attacks can be life-threatening. Appropriate medication is necessary during an acute attack. A peak-flow meter should be used to monitor breathing.

 ## Nutritional and Herbal Therapies

NATURAL SUBSTANCES are available that can open constricted bronchial tubes without side effects. There are also natural therapies and other measures that can reduce the need for medication and the likelihood of an acute attack.

Researchers have known for half a century that magnesium sulfate acts as a natural bronchodilator that opens constricted bronchial tubes without adverse effects. Richard Firshein, D.O., director of the Firshein Center for Comprehensive Medicine in New York City, specializes in the treatment of asthma through natural and alternative therapies. He recommends 500 milligrams of magnesium aspartate daily. He observes that magnesium alone won't cure a severe attack, but intravenous magnesium sulfate can be given along with drugs by a trained practitioner to relax smooth muscle and rapidly open the bronchial tubes. Oral magnesium supplements are used for long-term maintenance. The Firshein asthma treatment protocol also includes licorice, ginkgo biloba, fish oil or flaxseed oil, organic foods, breathing exercises, and mind-body techniques.[41]

Asthma drugs have natural counterparts in the plant world. Alternative practitioners feel that using the whole plant provides a more balanced remedy and is less toxic than using just an extracted "active ingredient." Theophylline is found naturally in tea. It belongs to a group of drugs called xanthines that also includes caffeine (found in coffee) and theobromine (found in cocoa). Ephedrine's natural counterpart is herba ephedra, found in the grassy plant *ma huang,* used in Chinese medicine for thousands of years. Even cromolyn is new only to Western medicine. In the form of ammi seeds, it has been part of Bedouin folk medicine for centuries.[42]

The herb elecampane can help build up the lungs. Lung Complex by Enzymatic Therapy is an herbal formula that helps support the lungs.

Another herbal remedy good for relieving asthma symptoms is a gemmotherapy by Dolisos called Lithy Tree. The usual dose is twenty to forty drops once daily in two ounces of water, but for children with severe asthma, the dose can be repeated twice daily.

Alyce Giorgi, an herbalist in Southold, New York, reports permanent asthma cures with this simple home treatment: Slice a large Spanish onion and put it on the child's chest. Leave it for twenty to thirty minutes while the child breathes in the fumes. The eyes will tear, but the chest will open up. Giorgi asserts that she has seen cases in which children have thrown away their inhalers after this procedure was done only once.

Black-currant-seed oil is another natural remedy that opens the lungs for easier breathing. Useful for any type of breathing problem, it eases breathing by reducing inflammation in the lungs. The recommended dosage is two pills every morning. To relieve exercise-induced asthma, take two pills before workouts. For stress-induced asthma, try black currant gemmotherapy.

**Inhalers Avoided
with Black-Currant-Seed Oil**

Chloe, nineteen, had a long history of childhood asthma and recurring colds and chest infections. She wanted to attend college without constant illness and the need to rely on inhalers. A combination of homeopathic products, herbs, and black-currant-seed oil over approximately a year succeeded in clearing her problems. She is now off inhalers and doing well, and reports that she has not had a cold or lung problem in the last two years. She continues to take the black-currant-seed oil daily, increasing the dosage to two pills three to four times daily if she feels her lungs are getting "tight."

 Homeopathic Options

ASTHMA PLUS by Deseret and Asthma by BHI are remedies that support the lungs homeopathically. A German homeopathic remedy by Staufen called Asthma is also quite effective.

Homeopaths feel that many cases of asthma are caused by suppressed pneumonia (pneumonia that has been treated by antibiotics). In these cases, Staufen series therapy (available in the United States from Deseret) is very effective. Consult a homeopath.

For allergic asthma caused by cockroaches, the appropriate homeopathic remedy is Blatta 6x or 30x taken three times daily.

For dust-mite allergies, Biting Insects by Molecular Biologicals can help.

> ## Steroid Side Effects Avoided with Homeopathic Remedies
>
> Vincent was described by his mother as a kind and loving child until steroids were prescribed for his asthma at the age of four. Suddenly, she said, he became a "brat"—hyperactive, belligerent, rude, climbing the walls. This behavior went on for nearly a year, until she got homeopathic advice and began giving Vincent a homeopathic remedy in place of the drugs. He was then able to engage in sports without wheezing, yet remained calm, cheerful, and polite. "I got my boy back," she said.

 ## The Approach of Chinese Medicine

ACUPUNCTURE CAN also help alleviate asthma. A Chinese study published in 1989 reported a disappearance or decreased frequency of asthma attacks in 88.9 percent of cases treated by a particular acupuncture method.[43] Rings are available from acupuncturists that have proven effective in quelling asthma attacks. They are slid up and down on the fingers, stimulating the acupuncture points on the hands and balancing the body.

Two common causes of asthma, according to Chinese medicine, are "cold in the lungs" and suppressed anger or grief. The typical childhood case involves parental death or divorce. Within a short time, the child begins to have lung problems—coughing, congestion in the morning, frequent colds and flu, which may turn into pneumonia or bronchitis. Homeopathic remedies like Ignatia 200x can help release this "grief trapped in the lungs."

Other Nondrug Alternatives

EXERCISE IS a natural adrenaline stimulant. Teaching the child to breathe properly from the diaphragm and to empty the lungs completely on exhalation is also important.[44] Karate or yoga classes could help in this pursuit.

F. Batmanghelidj, M.D., in *Your Body's Many Cries for Water,* reports some remarkable asthma cures with water therapy. He states we need half our body's weight in ounces of water per day—not soft drinks, juices, coffee, or tea, but plain (filtered or bottled) water. Thus a child weighing sixty-four pounds would need thirty-two ounces, or four glasses, daily. Wait half an hour before meals and two and a half hours after meals to take these heavy water doses, to avoid diluting the digestive juices.[45]

For other natural remedial and preventive approaches, and for dietary suggestions for asthma provoked by food allergies, see "Allergies." For substitutes for common allergenic foods, see "Nutrition."

ASTIGMATISM (See Vision Problems)

ATHLETE'S FOOT (See Fungal Infections)

ATTENTION DEFICIT HYPERACTIVITY DISORDER (ADD, ADHD)

ATTENTION DEFICIT hyperactivity disorder (ADHD) is a childhood condition characterized by an inability to concentrate, stay on task, or sit quietly. Also called minimal brain dysfunction, it is conventionally considered a form of brain damage, a diagnosis justifying treatment with drugs. The problem is that its symptoms can have many other causes. Studies have been unable to find consistent, objective evidence of the condition, which is not defined by a consistent cluster of symptoms.[46] According to the American Psychiatric Association, a child is considered to have ADHD when he shows eight of the following symptoms for at least six months, beginning before his seventh birthday: often fidgets his hands or feet or squirms in his seat; has trouble staying in his seat when required; is easily distracted; has trouble waiting his turn; often blurts out answers before a question is completed; has trouble doing chores or otherwise following through with instructions; has trouble sustaining attention to work or play activities; often shifts from one unfinished task to another; has trouble playing quietly; often talks too much; often interrupts others or butts in on other children's games; doesn't seem to listen to what's being said; often loses things (toys, pencils, books, assignments); does dangerous things without considering the consequences, like running into the street without looking.[47]

The vagueness of these criteria has led to obvious problems in categorization, since most children display some of these traits. The younger a child is, the more difficult diagnosing mental disorder becomes. Children under six do not express themselves well, their brains and behavior are changing rapidly, and they are very reactive to their environments.[48] Vagueness in diagnosis, in turn, has led to serious problems with treatment. Millions of children may be on powerful amphetamines unnecessarily. The drugs merely mask symptoms without addressing the cause, while compounding the problem with side effects.

 ## Conventional Treatment

RITALIN (METHYLPHENIDATE) is the most popular conventional treatment for ADHD. A powerful amphetamine, Ritalin is classified as a schedule II drug, a category that includes opium and morphine. Ritalin belongs to a family of drugs that stimulate the central nervous system and increase alertness and the ability to pay attention. It carries the warning that it "should not be used in children under six years, since safety and efficacy in this age group have not been established." Despite that warning, according to a report in the February 2000 *Journal of the American Medical Association,* an acute increase has occurred in the number of preschoolers taking Ritalin, Prozac, and other psychotropic drugs.[49]

Ritalin's side effects are like those of other amphetamines: sleeplessness, loss of appetite, irritability, headaches, fatigue, withdrawal, crying for no apparent reason, and a sensitivity to criticism that resembles depression. There may also be a stunting of growth. One of the most serious potential side effects is the development of tics—involuntary, darting, purposeless motor movements of the face or arms. The tics can progress to Tourette's syndrome, a condition characterized by generalized jerking movements in any part of the body, accompanied by a tendency to use foul language and repeat words.[50] These side effects have led to a spate of lawsuits on behalf of children allegedly harmed by inappropriate use of the drug. Ritalin has also caused cancer in mice; the FDA warning states that "the significance of these results to humans is unknown."

 Finding the Cause

THE FIRST step in a holistic approach to ADHD is to determine the condition's cause. Possibilities include reading or other learning disabilities, problems at home, problems at school (ineffective teaching or boring subject matter), nutritional deficiencies, low blood sugar, food allergies, buried emotional trauma, toxic chemical poisoning, and parasites. Hay fever is another potential cause of irritability, mood swings, and insomnia. The drugs used to treat this environmental allergy can make victims drowsy and slow. The result can be a short attention span, difficulty learning, and disruptive behavior in school.[51] (See "Allergies.")

ADD Traced to Toxoplasmosis and Eliminated

A mother who had been treated for parasites and had gotten significant relief mentioned that her ten-year-old daughter was having problems at school: The girl slept a lot and wasn't very active. Within two weeks of taking remedies for parasites, the girl "came alive" again. She soon began getting straight A's, had more friends, felt much better, and was more active. Both mother and daughter had toxoplasmosis, a parasitic infection acquired from cats. The mother may have had it while pregnant. It had evidently settled in the child's brain so she couldn't think clearly.

 Nutritional Approaches

AUTHOR DR. SMITH found in his practice that nutritional supplementation alone could control the unacceptable behavior of hyperactive children by 60 to 90 percent. Hair analyses showed these children to be low in both magnesium and calcium, although they were drinking sufficient quantities of milk. Magnesium is necessary for the enzyme that makes a brain chemical in which hyperactive children are deficient. About three weeks of supplementation with 500 milligrams of magnesium and 1,000 milligrams of calcium daily helped rebuild depleted supplies. Calcium and magnesium can also help alleviate the sleep disorders associated with ADHD (or the amphetamines taken for it). Other nutritional modifications Dr. Smith found to help included 50 milligrams of vitamin B_6 (if dream recall was poor), omitting dairy foods from the diet (if ear infections were a problem in infancy), and supplementing with essential fatty acids (if dry skin or eczema was a problem).

Studies have found that children with ADHD tend to have low levels of the omega-3 fatty acids necessary for normal brain and nervous system development. This is not genetic—it is the result of eating too much junk food. Most convenience foods are high in trans fatty acids, the highly processed kind that interferes with normal fat metabolism. Unbalanced diets heavy in sugar and junk food rob the brain of the raw materials it needs for the neurotransmitters that control brain function.[52] Omega-3 fatty acids can be obtained by eating fish or by taking fish oil supplements. Another option is a product called Attention Focus, which is designed specifically for the dietary management of fatty acid deficiency in ADD or ADHD. The recommended dose for children over five years old is four capsules twice daily with food or drink for the first twelve weeks. For younger children, the dose is reduced to two or three capsules twice daily. Child Life also makes a product called Essential Fatty Acids that comes in liquid form and is easy for kids to take.

For ADD-like learning problems, DMAE (dimethylaminoethanol) and PS (phosphatidylserine) may also help.[53] A product called Pedi-Active ADD contains DMAE, PS, and phosphatidylcholine in chewable tablet form. The dose is two tablets three times daily. Pedi-Active also comes in a bar form that can be sent in school lunch boxes.

Pycnogenol, a powerful antioxidant derived from French maritime pine trees, is also reported to help in cases of ADHD. An appropriate childhood dose is 50 milligrams daily.

For children who have trouble with dream recall, pyridoxine may help.

 ## The Food Allergy Factor

FOOD ALLERGIES are another potential cause of hyperactivity. In a study reported by allergist and pediatrician William Crook, M.D., of over one hundred children, the condition was traced to food allergies in about three-fourths of them. In a study conducted at London's Institute of Child Health and Hospital for Sick Children, twenty-eight hyperactive children were fed one of two selected foods, each for one week.

The suspect food was associated with symptoms in the child; the control food wasn't. Dramatic improvement in behavior was noted during the week the control food was eaten.

Likely allergens include cow's milk, wheat, corn, yeast, soy, sugar, citrus fruits or juices, chocolate, eggs, nuts, fish, and berries. If you suspect a food allergy in your child, try eliminating possible offenders, then adding them back into the diet one by one. If a food is definitely implicated by the return of symptoms, eliminate it from the diet for at least three months, then have the child try it cautiously. If no reaction occurs, it can be eaten in moderation.[54]

The late Ben Feingold, M.D., chief of the allergy clinics of the Kaiser Foundation in California, linked hyperactivity not only to foods but to food additives and chemicals, including those in Ritalin itself. A New York study reported in 1994 found that nineteen of twenty-six children with ADHD were sensitive to certain foods, dyes, or preservatives.[55]

 Mental and Emotional Factors

EVEN IF the problem is in fact mental or emotional, there are solutions that are both safer than drugs and more effective over the long term. Children often improve as dramatically with attention from their families or their school as they do on Ritalin.[56] For specific learning disabilities, tutoring or remedial reading classes are available. If the problem is social or psychological, counseling is recommended.

For emotional trauma, homeopathic remedies and Rescue Remedy, a Bach flower remedy, can help. Aromatherapy is also calming and relaxing. Chamomile oil is good for the child who has trouble relaxing or is hyperactive, nervous, or upset. Try putting lavender oil in the bedroom, by or on the child's pillow or on a rag placed near the bed, or burn a lavender-scented candle in the room. Pillows with lavender seeds are also available.

Hyperactivity Traced to Childhood Trauma and Eliminated

An adopted girl of six or seven was hyperactive and would not go to sleep until her mother had stayed by her bed for several hours each night. If the girl awoke and her mother wasn't there, she screamed and became hysterical. Rescue Remedy, along with an antimiasmatic homeopathic remedy called Multiple Miasm by Deseret, made a remarkable difference in her. The girl began telling her mother of dreams and memories of her early years with her natural parents, who had abused her. Multiple Miasm is said to revive old memories, bringing them to consciousness. They can then be cleared so that they are no longer suppressed in and suppressing the system. The mother was thrilled with the changes in the girl, who seemed to have matured by four or five years in six months. The child would finally sleep alone and could fall immediately to sleep.

Toxic Chemical Buildup and ADD

ANOTHER POSSIBLE cause of hyperactivity is toxic-chemical and heavy-metal poisoning. Whether the symptoms of ADD and ADHD are caused or merely aggravated by toxic residues in the system, homeopathic detoxification remedies can be useful adjuncts. Behavioral symptoms are worsened by the buildup of toxins and are improved by reducing their levels in the body. Childhood autism, which is conventionally considered irreversible, has been reversed in several cases by chelation to remove heavy metals. Homeopathic remedies are also available for detoxifying heavy metals. (See "Heavy-metal Poisoning.")

ADD Traced to Pesticide Poisoning and Eliminated

A nine-year-old Boise, Idaho, boy with ADD was on major antidepressants and antipsychotic medications after he had gone through all the usual medicines, including Ritalin, without getting better. Investigation revealed that he lived in an area that had been heavily sprayed in the sixties and seventies with paraquat, a highly toxic pesticide. He was given homeopathic remedies for detoxification, including a German formula specifically for paraquat poisoning, and products called Addiclenz and Enviroclenz by Deseret. (See "Environmental Illness.")

The process was very difficult for the boy, and the detox had to be done slowly. He was started at one drop a day, working up to ten drops over a long period of time. When his system was finally cleared of the toxic chemical, his delighted mother reported dramatic improvement. He was much calmer; no longer got depressed, suicidal, or angry; and no longer picked on other kids.

AUTISM

AUTISM IS a baffling condition in which children are withdrawn and unable to communicate normally, although they can be bright in other ways. They seem to be responding to their own inner world. They have no eye contact with parents or other children and often engage in self-stimulating activity like rocking or waving their hands in purposeless movements. Autism is usually apparent soon after birth but at least by age three. A few decades ago the condition was blamed on a mother's failure to rock or hold the child, who then turned to self-stimulation; but new evidence has shifted blame to the drug and chemical industries.

Suggested causal factors include lead poisoning, infant vaccinations, food additives including aspartame and food dyes, and overuse of antibiotics for ear infections. Antibiotics wipe out friendly bacteria in the gut, allowing an overgrowth of yeast resulting in candida infections, autoimmune reactions, and food allergies, all of which are commonly found in autistic children. Other possible causes include fetal alcohol syndrome, viral infections, and parasites.[57]

Dr. Bernard Rimland, founding director of the Autism Research Institute, blames childhood vaccine programs for the epidemic of childhood autism. There are now a minimum of two hundred and fifty thousand autistic children in the United States, a ten- to fifteen-fold increase since immunization came into vogue. The suspect MMR (measles/mumps/rubella) vaccine is first incubated in chick-embryo culture. The concern is that the virus becomes programmed to produce antibodies against the protein of the myelin sheath of the chick and then of the child. Childhood autism is caused by encephalitis (brain inflammation) affecting the limbic system of the brain.

Heredity also seems to be a factor. Recent studies suggest that vaccines and other toxic environmental insults may trigger a genetic predisposition toward physiological abnormalities in the intestinal, immune, and neurological systems of certain infants. In a study of autistic children recently conducted at Oregon Health Sciences University in Portland, Oregon, nearly all the children studied had family histories of autism, attention deficit, developmental delays, and various mental abnormalities, usually involving communication deficits. Significant improvements in the children's conditions resulted when they were put on casein- and gluten-free diets with added nutrients, and were given antifungals (natural or prescription) and probiotics (acidophilus made from whey to aid in the reduction of yeast) and/or secretin, a digestive enzyme.

For further information on autism, contact the Autism Research Institute in San Diego, directed by Dr. Bernard Rimland, 619-281-7165; the Autism Services Center, 304-525-8014; or the Autism Society of America, 301-565-0433.

Conventional Treatment

CONVENTIONAL TREATMENT for autism is aimed at keeping the child calm and controlled, either with drugs, behavior modification, or institutionalization. There is no conventional cure for the disease.

Natural Alternative Treatment

ALTERNATIVE TREATMENT has reported some cures. For a remarkable series of cases involving lead poisoning that were reversed with chelation, see "Heavy-metal Poisoning."

Nutritional supplementation, dietary regulation, craniosacral therapy, and auditory integration training may also help relieve the symptoms of autism. Megavitamin therapy emphasizes vitamin B_6, magnesium, vitamin C, and dimethylglycine (DMG). Dietary approaches involve locating and avoiding allergenic foods (milk, gluten-containing products, sugar, corn, and eggs are likely suspects) and toxic additives (food dyes, aspartame, etc.). The digestive enzyme secretin has also been used, but routine intravenous injection (usually once every four to six weeks) over a long period of time seems to be required for it to have a significant effect.

Craniosacral therapy can reduce or eliminate erratic behavior like head banging, apparently by relieving cranial restrictions that distort the brain. Craniosacral therapy is a technique based on cranial osteopathy taught by the International Association of Health Care Practitioners in Palm Beach Gardens, Florida, headed by John Upledger, D.O. It works with the rhythm in the cranial system that results from the increase and decrease in volume of the cerebrospinal fluid. The craniosacral rhythm causes the skull bones to move in a slight but predictable way. Restrictions to this movement can result from the birthing process. Craniosacral manipulation releases these restrictions and restores function.

For children who display autistic behavior after receiving the DPT (diphtheria/pertussis/tetanus) or MMR vaccines, a blood titer test may be useful. If a high titer is present for any of these inoculations, immune-globulin injections will sometimes help lower it.

Auditory integration training deals with the highly sensitive hearing of autistic children, which can make them afraid of sounds and people and can block their ability to concentrate. Training is done with music or the filtered sounds of the mother's voice. For more information, contact the Georgiana Organization, 203-454-1221, or the Sound, Listening and Learning Center, 602-381-0086.

For specific behavioral problems in autistic children, homeopathic remedies may help.

Autistic Child's Behavior Improves with Homeopathy

A mother brought her severely autistic fourteen-year-old daughter to author Dr. Walker, complaining of a relatively new array of symptoms involving pinching, biting, and holding her stomach. Questioning revealed that these symptoms were worse around the full moon, a giveaway clue to parasitic infestation, since worms lay their eggs then. The girl was given the homeopathic remedy Worms by CompliMed, and within two weeks the symptoms had gone away. (See "Parasites.") While she had stopped biting and punching and was much more pleasant, she still had one problematic symptom: She would drop her head back and go into seizure-like behavior. Dr. Walker gave the girl Tarentula, a constitutional homeopathic remedy specific for her particular personality and symptom complex. Following this treatment, the mother was delighted to report that her daughter had gone out for the first time ever and played by herself for half an hour. Before that, she would not leave her mother's side. The girl also became calmer, happier, and no longer has seizurelike behavior.

BAD MOODS (See Anger)

BED-WETTING (ENURESIS)

ENURESIS IS the persistent emptying of the bladder during sleep. Normal in babies, it is considered problematic after about four years of age in girls or five years of age in boys; 15 percent of boys and 8 percent of girls suffer from it. The syndrome has been ascribed to a variety of causes, including emotional upsets, a small bladder, and too many fluids near bedtime.

 Home Treatment

MOST BED-WETTING problems can be resolved by taking one or more of the following measures:

1. Allow nothing sugary at bedtime. Instead, substitute a protein food to keep the blood sugar from falling during the night. When the blood sugar falls, the brain does not respond as well to the bladder's message of fullness, allowing the child to sleep through this signal.

2. Give 500 milligrams of magnesium at bedtime to help the bladder relax, expand, and hold more urine during the night.

3. If the child has had persistent ear infections, tonsillitis, or phlegm, a cow's-milk sensitivity is likely. These children should avoid milk products after lunchtime, since they can irritate sensitive bladders and cause night emptying.

4. Chiropractic adjustments of the neck or pelvis have been known to help in some cases.

5. Children who are simply very deep sleepers may respond to a wired device that reacts to a urine leak by ringing a bell. The bell helps condition the child to respond to the full-bladder sensation. While these children may be such deep sleepers that the device awakens only the parents, it is worth a try.

Homeopathic remedies for bed-wetting include Hyland's bed-wetting tablets, Uri-control by BHI, and homeopathic Equisetum 6x or 30x, given before bedtime.

Homeopathic Remedy Gives Quick Results

Jay suddenly began wetting his bed at the age of five. His parents had tried a number of solutions to no avail and were at their wits' end. They were delighted when Uri-control given at bedtime halted the problem in about four days.

BEE STINGS (See Insect Bites)

BLADDER INFECTION (CYSTITIS)

CYSTITIS, OR bladder infection, is far more common in girls than boys, since girls' urethras are shorter and close to the anus and vagina. Symptoms of bladder infection include frequency of urination, a sense of urgency, painful burning, and sometimes bleeding. Before local symptoms are apparent, children with bladder infections may have fever and malaise (weakness and listlessness). Most bladder infections are caused by the bacteria *Escherichia coli*, normally found in the intestines. Improper wiping (from back to front) is a likely route of infection. Less common causes of recurring bladder infections are bubble baths and sexual abuse.

Drug Treatment

ANTIBIOTICS ARE the usual treatment for cystitis, following a culture to determine which antibiotics are sensitive to the urine. For antibiotic downsides, see "Immunity."

Homeopathic and Herbal Remedies

HOMEOPATHIC DOCTORS maintain that antibiotics don't cure urinary tract infections but merely suppress their symptoms. Homeopathic remedies draw the problem to the surface and help the body eliminate it. For bladder infections, homeopathic Cantharis is excellent. The recommended dosage for treating intense burning before, during, and after urination is three pellets of Cantharis 6x or 30c four times daily. Sarsaparilla 6c to 30c is also effective. The dosage is three pellets four times daily.

These single homeopathic remedies work at the onset of a bladder infection (the first or second day), but after the problem has gone on for several days, a combination of homeopathic and herbal remedies is more effective. Use either Tao Chin Pien (a Chinese herbal combination) or Bacticin or Cystimed by CompliMed, along with Bladder Irritation by Natra-Bio or Uri-Control by BHI, following these schedules:

* Bacticin or Cystimed: ten drops every fifteen minutes for the first hour, then once an hour for four hours, then four times daily until the infection is completely gone.

* Uri-Control: one tablet every hour for the first four hours, then one tablet four times daily.

Nutritional Remedies

BECAUSE BACTERIA are more likely to multiply in alkaline urine, keeping the urine acidic usually helps. Cranberry juice, an old-wives' remedy for bladder infections, has been shown in clinical studies to actually reduce cystitis pain and recurrences. The juice acidifies the urine, inhibiting bacterial growth, and engulfs the infecting bacteria to prevent them from becoming attached to the cells lining the urinary tract. To achieve this result, use only the pure juice: "Cocktails" can contain as little as 2 percent juice. The bitter cranberry taste can be alleviated with cold seltzer or sweeteners, or add a teaspoon of pure juice to a cup of tea. Uva ursi, a type of cranberry, can also be made into tea; or you can buy cranberry capsules.

Cranberry Emer'gen-C, an effervescent vitamin C with cranberry by Alacer, is good for bladder infections, and children love the fizzy effervescence.

A combination of parsley and celery juices (fresh-squeezed) acts as a natural diuretic that flushes the body. Avoid citrus juices, which can irritate the bladder.

If antibiotics are used, always follow them with acidophilus to replace friendly intestinal flora. Acidophilus supplements are more effective than yogurt. (See "Candidiasis.") PB-8 by Nutrition Now is a good product for kids. It contains eight different types of acidophilus in powdered form. The same company also makes flavored chewable acidophilus tablets.

Copious amounts of water (preferably distilled) should be drunk daily to flush out the bladder, dilute toxins, and prevent bacteria from going back up the urethra and infecting the kidneys.

Other Helpful Tips

* Teach the child to wipe from front to rear.

* Encourage frequent emptying of the bladder. Holding the urine can increase bladder infections.

* Underwear should have cotton crotches.

* Hot tubs should be avoided.

* Teenage girls should change sanitary napkins frequently (and tampons if used; but they are best avoided, since they hold toxins in the body and are linked to toxic shock syndrome).

BLOODY NOSE (See Nosebleeds)

BODY PIERCING (See Skin Infections)

BOILS (See Skin Infections)

BONES, BROKEN OR FRACTURED

BROKEN BONES may be quite obvious when they occur in an arm or leg, but hairline fractures may cause only some pain and slight swelling. All need professional care. The patient should be transported with suitable splinting to a hospital or doctor's office. If a fracture is suspected, careful X rays should be taken, since the bones need to be properly positioned while healing. The obvious bone deformities should be splinted without any attempt to manipulate them: "Splint them where they lie." Perhaps the most effective splinting method that can be done at home is to use a rolled-up newspaper, blanket, or pillow to softly support the break. Careful splinting prevents a simple fracture from becoming compound; that is, having the bone end push through the skin, a condition that may result in infection and complicate healing.

A *rib fracture,* or broken rib, is common after a direct blow to the chest, as from falls on objects or from car accidents. X rays are usually not indicated in simple cases. Taping the chest has long been the standard treatment, but the muscles between the ribs can hold the rib ends in the right position for healing without this procedure; and while an elastic bandage around the chest might help to control the pain associated with breathing, if the breathing is constricted unduly, patients can develop pneumonia from insufficient aeration of the lungs. Analgesics are suggested to control pain.

 Homeopathic Treatment

THE NORMAL healing time for a broken bone is about seven weeks. However, the homeopathic remedy Symphytum 6c or 30c (three pills, three times a day) has been known to shorten this time to a week or two. Homeopathic Arnica can prevent the body from overreacting to trauma.

Doctor Amazed at Rapid Bone Healing

A mother sought help for her nine-year-old son who had broken his leg skiing in Sun Valley, where author Dr. Walker had a practice and an herb shop. The boy's leg was in a cast, which his doctor said would have to remain in place for at least two months. However, two and a half weeks after the boy began taking Symphytum, the doctor x-rayed the leg and removed the cast. He remarked that he couldn't believe how fast the bone had healed. Dr. Walker frequently saw this sort of rapid healing of broken legs with Symphytum while she was in Sun Valley.

BOWEL CONTROL (See Toilet Training)

BOWLEGS

BOWLEGS IS a condition in which the legs are bent like a cowboy's around a horse. Decades ago, when rickets was common, bowlegs appeared when a child whose bones were insufficiently calcified began to walk and his weight bent the bones. We now know rickets is caused by a deficiency of vitamin D, which is necessary for the absorption of calcium. The condition is easily treated with vitamin D or sunshine, the most ubiquitous source of the vitamin. Most cow's-milk formulas are fortified with vitamin D. Human milk usually contains enough of it without fortification, but vitamin-D drops are still a good precautionary measure.

BREAST-FEEDING

THAT BREAST milk is the best food for human babies is no longer in dispute. The American Academy of Pediatrics recommends that full-term infants be breast-fed exclusively. The most important period is the first four to six months of life. Breast-feeding provides substantial benefits in nutrition as well as bone structure and improved immunity. Even intelligence has been shown to be enhanced, apparently by the essential fatty acids present in mother's milk. Breast-fed babies have fewer episodes of ear infection, respiratory infection, and meningitis.[58]

Breast-feeding also helps the facial bones develop properly, since the breast-fed baby must open his or her mouth wide enough to squeeze the milk-containing lacteal glands (under the edge of the areolar border of the nipple, where the darker color ends). This stretching exercises the mouth and allows the facial bones to grow enough to achieve their full potential. Children who have been breast-fed for close to a year are more likely to have evenly spaced teeth and well-constructed dental arches in their later years and are less likely to need orthodontia.

If the nursing mother eats a good diet, her milk will have all the amino acids, sugars, fats, and other nutrients the baby needs for growth and brain development. Solid foods are unnecessary for babies and may even cause food sensitivities the infant never outgrows. (For solid-food feeding schedules, see "Nutrition.")

Early cow's-milk feeding may also cause food sensitivities. While the American Academy of Pediatrics states that only about 5 percent of Americans are allergic to cow's milk,[59] clinical observation suggests that many more are sensitive to it, and the early use of cow's-milk formula may be largely to blame. Pediatricians routinely switch babies from cow's milk to goat's milk or meat-based formula when babies have colic, a rash, or vomiting. The same cow's-milk sensitivity can lead to ear infections, asthma, bed-wetting, headaches, swollen tonsils and adenoids, and general susceptibility to infections. Too-early feeding of cow's milk has also been linked to type 1 diabetes, a condition that leads to a lifelong need for insulin.[60] (See "Diabetes.")

The breast-feeding mother should check her own diet not only for proper nutrients but for allergenic foods. A baby may have what appears to be an allergic reaction to breast milk, when he or she is actually reacting to some food the mother ate to which the baby is sensitive. Likely offenders include dairy, garlic, nuts, eggs, and corn. However, food sensitivities are very individual and there are many other possibilities.

Colostrum, the first mammary secretion of lactating animals and humans, contains immune-building factors that bottle-fed babies miss. Colostrum from cows can now be purchased in supplement form to build the immunity of bottle-fed babies. It can also be given to children to prevent or relieve the symptoms of colds or flu. For a discussion of nutritional supplements in general, see "Nutrition."

 ## Natural Remedies for Nursing Difficulties

AS SOON after birth as possible, babies should be allowed to latch on to their mothers' breasts. If they are not able to open their mouths sufficiently to place their gums on the edge of the areolar border of the nipple and empty the breasts, feeding may be insufficient. If the baby's mouth cannot open wide enough to accommodate about three of his or her fingers, a temporomandibular joint (jaw) dysfunction may have occurred from the tumultuous ordeal of delivery. A craniosacral therapist, osteopathic physician, or chiropractor can do a cranial adjustment to relieve this problem and allow the baby to nurse.

For problems with lactation, homeopathic remedies can help. Here are some alternatives for specific conditions:

Chinchona 30c: for fatigue due to breast-feeding

Urtica urens 30c: for an insufficient supply of milk

Pulsatilla 30c: for an overabundant milk supply or to decrease supply

Ricinus 30c: to stop milk supply altogether when weaning

Phellandrium 9c: for relief if breast-feeding is painful (three pellets ten minutes before breast-feeding)

Hepar sulph: for a minor abscess in the breast

Belladonna: for the early stages of an abscess in the breast, when the skin is red and hot

Bryonia: for mastitis

Graphites: for cracks around the nipples; homeopathic calendula cream may also be used topically

To relieve painful engorgement, the mother should persist in nursing until the baby drains the milk from her breast.

Mastitis Relieved with Natural Remedy

A young mother with severely cracked nipples and mastitis was given Bryonia orally along with Calendula lotion for topical application to the nipple. After only one day of treatment, she was pleased to report that the problem was nearly cured.

BREATH-HOLDING (See Anger)

BRONCHITIS

BRONCHITIS, OR inflammation of the bronchioles of the lungs, is most commonly attributed to a virus, although secondary bacterial infections are fairly common. Acute bronchitis may follow a cold and involves coughing up a thick green or yellow mucus. It lasts about a week. A sensitivity to cow's milk can trigger the condition by thickening mucus secretions, creating a fertile field in which microbes can grow.

Conventional Treatment

BRONCHITIS CAUSED by bacteria is conventionally treated with antibiotics. For downsides, see "Immunity." Viral bronchitis clears up without drug treatment.

 Natural Alternatives

HERBS USEFUL in relieving bronchitis include ephedra, eucalyptus leaf, ginger root, horehound, ivy leaf, and thyme.

Vitamin C can be given in doses of up to 1,000 milligrams every two to four hours along with echinacea at the beginning of the illness; but the echinacea should be discontinued thereafter, as it can actually hold germs in the lungs. (See "Colds.")

European Filbert by Dolisos is a gemmotherapy good for relieving the symptoms of bronchitis.

Chinese patent herbal remedies are also available. When there is deep phlegm in the chest and a rattling cough tending toward bronchitis, the remedy is Ping Chuan, ten pills twice daily. For full-fledged bronchitis with a cough and deep rattles in the chest, the remedy is Hsiao Keh Chuan, two pills, three times daily. This formula also comes in the form of a cough syrup.

Old-fashioned mustard plasters can be quite effective in relieving congestion in the chest, either from chronic lung infection that won't clear, a cold that is "stuck" in the chest, or backaches caused by lung congestion. The mustard plaster pulls the heat to the surface of the skin and loosens congestion, bringing significant relief to the child. For a small child, use one teaspoon of dried mustard, four tablespoons of flour, and one teaspoon of oil. For a larger chest area, double the amounts of mustard and oil. Mix in lukewarm water to form a paste, spread the paste on half of a thin clean cloth, and fold over the other half to cover the paste mixture. Rub castor oil on the child's chest, then put a tight-fitting T-shirt on him and put him to bed. Place the plaster on the chest under the T-shirt, securing with pins if necessary. A heating pad or hot water bottle can be placed over the T-shirt for extra heat. Leave on for twenty to sixty minutes, less for a child under four. Check the skin regularly for heat; leaving mustard on too long can burn the skin, particularly if using an external heat source. You can cover the child's head and chest with a sheet so that he breathes the fumes.

For children prone to repeated bronchial infections, modify the diet to limit mucus-forming foods. Cow's milk is the chief offender. White flour products are also mucus-forming. For dietary substitutes for milk and wheat, see "Nutrition."

For other natural remedies, see "Colds."

BRUISES (See Trauma)

BULIMA (See Anorexia)

BURNS

BURNS ARE common in children, who are prone to putting their hands on the burners of stoves or spilling hot liquids onto themselves. For burned fingers, the best emergency treatment is to plunge the fingers into cold water and hold them there for a few minutes (ice water was once recommended for this purpose, but cold water is equally effective). Petroleum jelly, an over-the-counter product commonly used on burns, is not recommended because it actually holds in the heat; it is like "boiling in oil." This is also true for butter, an old home remedy.

Natural Alternatives

ALOE VERA has produced amazing results on burns, especially when the fresh plant is used. The procedure is to cut open the plant and simply apply it directly to the burn. Aloe vera has been known to heal even severe burns in just a day or two if applied immediately. Many people keep an aloe plant in the house or yard for just such emergencies. Creams and liniments containing aloe vera are also available commercially.

Homeopathic Cantharis and Causticum are other effective remedies for burns and sunburn.

For electric-shock burns, the homeopathic remedy is Electricity 200x.

For severe burns, high doses of vitamin C (one to two grams daily) have been shown to speed healing.

CANDIDIASIS, THRUSH

FUNGI ARE the most common parasites, led by the ubiquitous yeast *Candida albicans*. Candida produces lesions called thrush in the mouth, gluteal folds, neck, groin, and armpits. Thrush can appear as a bright or dark red diaper rash that doesn't respond to ointments for ordinary rash. Yeast diaper rashes are usually worst in warm, damp skin folds. Thrush can also appear as white patches that leave red sores in the mouth.

Candidiasis can be acquired by the newborn when passing through the birth canal; from a mother with a vaginal infection; or when nursing, from a mother with a nipple infection. It may also follow a course of antibiotics. Candida organisms are natural residents of the body but are normally found in harmless proportions. The body's natural defense against fungus infection is its resident population of normal bacterial flora, which prevents invasion by foreigners. When antibiotics wipe out friendly along with unfriendly bacteria, the field is left wide open for this yeast to move in. See also "Fungal Infections."

For toxic reactions to black mold, another form of fungus, see "Environmental Illness."

 ## Conventional Treatment

FOR TOPICAL use on diaper rash and vaginal yeast infections, miconazole or clotrimazole (Lotrimin, GyneLotrimin, Lotrisone) may be used. These nonprescription drugs are considered relatively safe, but allergic reactions, irritation, burning, and stinging can occur. Nystatin (mycostatin) is also used topically for local yeast infections or as a gargle in the mouth. This is another nonprescription drug that is relatively safe, but it can produce nausea, vomiting, and diarrhea.

Nonprescription drugs don't work on more serious systemic (whole-body) fungal infections. For their treatment, the likely candidate until recently was amphotericin B, a toxic drug that has to be injected and can seriously damage the kidneys. Today Diflucan (fluconazole) is recommended, since it has fewer short-term side effects and can be taken orally. However, the standard drug reference *1998 Drug Facts and Comparisons* indicates that it, too, can have insidious long-term side effects, including a remote but real risk of serious liver damage.

 ## The Alternative Approach

CANDIDA INVASION typically results after an antibiotic, steroid, or other drug has suppressed the immune system, allowing the fungus to grow. Treatment aimed at killing the fungus is an imperfect solution, since the fungus can return when the drug is stopped. Some practitioners recommend special diets that eliminate foods on which candida feeds, but these diets are also imperfect solutions, since candida returns when sugar or fermented foods are eaten again.

Homeopaths feel that candida overgrowth is just a signal that the immune system is not working properly, due to overexposure to antibiotics or other drugs, or to environmental toxins. Antibiotics merely push the bacteria deeper, suppressing the immune system and allowing candida to grow. The homeopathic approach is to use remedies that boost the immune system so the body stops the fungus from multiplying. Good homeopathic formulas that address the cause of fungal invasion include Mycocan Combo by PHP (ten drops, three times daily), Candida Plus and FNG by Deseret, and Fungisode by Molecular Biologicals. Aquaphase is a candida swish-and-swallow wash.

Certain herbs and nutrients also have antifungal properties; garlic is one. In laboratory experiments, its antifungal activity has been shown to be greater than that of either nystatin or amphotericin B.[61] Health food stores now sell deodorized garlic tablets that make this age-old remedy both easy to take and socially acceptable. Garlic has been used in poultices, but it should not be used on babies' bottoms because it can irritate.[62]

Other useful herbal and nutritional antimicrobials include grapefruit-seed extract (NutriBiotic or ProSeed), olive-leaf extract, barberry, Pau d'Arco (a South American anti-infective herb), caprylic acid (a medium-chain fatty acid found naturally in the body that counters microorganism growth), undecylenic acid (another fat found naturally in the body, produced commercially from castor-bean oil), and oregano.

A combination product incorporating many of these herbs that is easy and convenient to use is Candistroy by Nature's Secret. Recommended for people over sixteen, it contains a variety of herbs that fight candida and boost the immune system, along with acidophilus.

Lactobacillus acidophilus, Bifidobacterium bifidum, and *Lactobacillus bulgaricus* are "good" bacteria that protect the digestive tract from invasion by unwanted microorganisms.[63] For children who have taken antibiotics, good bacteria should be replaced with these cultures. Some experts recommend yogurt, but not all yogurts contain live acidophilus cultures, and yogurt itself is a fermented food. Acidophilus supplements in liquid or capsule form are better. Child Life makes Friendly Flora/Bifidus for kids; PB-8 by Nutrition Now is another good product. It contains eight different types of acidophilus in powdered form. The same company also makes flavored chewable acidophilus tablets.

For natural remedies for vaginal yeast infections, see "Vaginitis."

 Other Helpful Tips

FOR BABIES with a yeast diaper rash, change diapers frequently, and immediately if wet or soiled. Clean the baby's bottom with plain water and allow to air-dry before rediapering. Allow air exposure as often as possible. Avoid plastic pants, which reduce air circulation.

An old-fashioned remedy for washing the bottom is witch hazel. Apple cider vinegar and lemon juice are other options for creating a more acid environment in which yeast are less able to grow. For soothing herbal remedies, see "Diaper Rash." Homeopathic Calendula lotion may also be applied topically.

For candidiasis in children old enough to eat solid foods, cut out fermented foods, mushrooms, yeast-containing foods, and moldy foods like blue cheese, vinegar, and pickles. Focus on pure, sugar-free foods. For creative alternatives, see *Get the Sugar Out* by Ann Louise Gittleman. For drinking, use bottled or purified water, not tap water.

Avoid using fabric softeners or scented detergent on underwear. Reduce exposure to toxic chemicals. Change damp socks or wet clothing, especially after perspiring.

Avoid the use of antibiotics unless critically necessary. Dairy products, which contain residues of the antibiotics given to dairy cows, can also make the situation worse and are best avoided. (See "Immunity.")

CANKER SORES (See Cold Sores)

CARBUNCLES (See Skin Infections)

CARIES (See Dental Problems)

CAR SICKNESS (See Nausea)

CAT SCRATCH DISEASE, BACILLARY ANGIOMATOSIS

CAT SCRATCH disease is a bacterial infection following a minor scratch by a cat (or dog), which can harbor infectious material in its claws. Symptoms include a low-grade fever and lymph node swellings. About two weeks usually elapse between the scratch and development of the skin lesion, which may drain pus. A newer form of cat scratch disease renamed *bacillary angiomatosis* has been reported in HIV-infected and other immune-compromised people.

 Conventional Treatment

ANTIBIOTICS MAY be prescribed for severe symptoms, but cat scratch disease does not respond well to antibiotics, which work poorly on this type of bacteria (gram-negative rods). Fortunately, the condition will heal by itself. Bacillary angiomatosis, the newer form of the disease, does respond to antibiotics (erythromycin).

Alternative Treatment

LEDUM IS the appropriate homeopathic remedy for these infections. Vitamin C and echinacea can also help shorten their course.

CELIAC DISEASE, GLUTEN INTOLERANCE

CELIAC DISEASE, characterized by chronic diarrhea, is a condition caused by insufficient intestinal enzymes to digest the glutens and carbohydrates found in wheat, rye, and other grains. The fermentation and putrefaction of these foods leads to frequent, greasy, foul-smelling stools.

Natural Solutions

THE CONDITION can be alleviated by taking digestive enzymes and avoiding gluten-containing foods. Gluten is found in wheat, barley, oats, and rye. It is also used as a filler in many prepared foods and medications. Check labels.

Homeopathic remedies are also available that can help relieve the condition. Possibilities include Lycopodium, Phosphorus, and Silicea.

CHARLEY HORSE (See Muscle Cramps, Pain, and Spasms)

CHICKEN POX

CHICKEN POX strikes more than three million children every year. It strikes only once, but the herpes zoster virus that causes it can become reactivated in adulthood as shingles, a much more serious disease. The symptoms of chicken pox consist of a red, itchy rash and fever. The rash is most common on the face, scalp, and chest but may also occur in the mouth. It consists of dark red papules on which blisters develop and then burst, forming scabs. The accompanying fever is usually mild and may be accompanied by fatigue and headache.

Chicken pox is extremely contagious, infecting 90 to 95 percent of exposed children who haven't yet had it. The disease takes about three weeks to incubate before flaring into visible pox, so many children are exposed to apparently healthy carriers. The carrier remains contagious from one to two days before the appearance of the rash until the pox are completely scabbed, with no new lesions for twenty-four hours. This generally takes about seven to ten days to occur. Children are advised to stay home from school until all of the blisters have crusted over.

 Drug Treatment

BECAUSE CHICKEN pox is rarely life-threatening and its first episode is a natural innoculation preventing future recurrences, researchers have been slow to develop a vaccine for it; but one finally hit the market in 1995. Critics point out that the duration of immune protection the vaccine provides is still unknown. Children may be better off acquiring a natural immunity in early childhood than putting off their first experience with the disease to a time when its symptoms are liable to be much more severe.[64] For other concerns about vaccines, see "Immunizations."

For relieving itching, calamine lotion applied topically remains the safest pharmaceutical option. Children enjoy applying this pink cream with a paintbrush.

To reduce the duration and severity of symptoms in serious cases of chicken pox, some doctors recommend acyclovir (Zovirax), a strong antiviral drug used for genital herpes. Acyclovir may also be recommended for a second case of chicken pox in the same household, which is likely to be more severe than the original case (evidently because the virus has had an opportunity to adapt and become more virulent). While the drug can reduce chicken pox symptoms, it can also expose the child to unnecessary side effects, including possible liver damage.[65]

Corticosteroids (cortisone) may also be used to treat chicken pox. These, too, are strong drugs with potentially serious side effects. They keep itching at bay by suppressing the immune system, but the immune system is the body's own weapon against infection (see "Itching"). Death in a recent chicken pox case was traced to the use of cortisone for an eye infection during the disease. The drug evidently suppressed the immune system so it could not fight the chicken pox virus.[66]

Oral antihistamines (for example, Benadryl) may be given when itchiness interferes with sleep. Antihistamines can also have side effects, but they are safer than corticosteroids.

For reducing fever, acetaminophen (Tylenol and others) is now generally recommended, since aspirin use by children with chicken pox or other viral illnesses has been linked to Reye's syndrome. (See "Reye's Syndrome.") However, some authorities question whether a normal fever should be reduced at all. In one study, children with chicken pox were given either acetaminophen or a placebo for four days. On the second day of treatment, children in the acetominophen-treated group were more active than those in the placebo group; but on the fourth day, the treated children itched more, and their chicken pox took a day longer to scab over. The data suggested that the effects of fever were actually beneficial in fighting off the virus, and that fever should be allowed to run its course.[67] (See "Fever.")

To relieve the pain of oral lesions, a simple oral solution made of equal parts Benadryl, antacid liquid, and teething gel may be recommended. It is swished in the mouth, then spit out.

Natural Alternatives

DAILY BATHS with baking soda or cornstarch (½ cup added to bathwater) can relieve itching naturally. Baths should be limited to once daily, since more can dry the skin and actually make it itchier. Ice applied directly to the itchiest pox can reduce swelling and discomfort. A fan over a bowl of ice, aimed at a particularly uncomfortable area, may also relieve itching.

A popular herbal remedy for drying up chicken pox and relieving itching is a tea tree oil cream applied directly to the skin. Another option is a vitamin A/D/E combination cream.

Calendula lotion or ointment helps soothe and heal any type of sore on the skin, from chicken pox to diaper rash. It should not, however, be used with homeopathic remedies because it contains camphor, which antidotes the remedies.

Clip fingernails and toenails and dress the child in loose-fitting clothes to help prevent scratching, which can leave permanent scars or lead to skin infections. After the pox have closed, scarring can be prevented with a natural product called ScarGo, containing olive oil, peanut oil, lanolin, camphor, and yellow beeswax.

For itching in the mouth, use a saltwater gargle.

For reducing fever, try the cold-water hip bath. Sit the child in just enough cold water to reach the hips, periodically swishing water over the stomach to cool it. Clay poultices applied to the stomach are also effective in relieving fever.

To reduce the dehydration that comes with fever, give plenty of fluids.

If given right when the pox break out, a homeopathic remedy for chicken pox called Varicella can make the case a very light one. Don't give Varicella before the breakout, since you want your child to develop an immunity to the virus.

Another homeopathic option is CompliMed's Cliniskin H, a combination of several remedies for chicken pox (Rhus tox, Cantharis,

Arsenicum alba, Mezereum). Give ten drops three to four times daily to speed drying of the pox and reduce irritability. A third homeopathic option is Viracin by CompliMed.

Chicken Pox Limited to Very Mild Case

The mother of a six-year-old boy was frantic when he was exposed to chicken pox at his day-care center, since she had to work and could not stay home with him. The boy was given the Staufen chicken pox remedy as soon as the pox started to break out. His relieved mother reported that he was sick for only a day and had just three pox, no fever, and none of the crying and misery that usually accompany the disease.

CIRCUMCISION

CIRCUMCISION IS the surgical amputation of some or all of the foreskin that covers the glans or head of the penis. The foreskin is a mobile sheath of skin containing sensitive nerve endings and a mucous membrane that covers and protects the glans, keeping it soft, moist, and sensitive.

Circumcision became commonplace in the United States in the nineteenth century, when it was believed the practice would stop masturbation and the spread of venereal disease. It did not prove to have these effects, and today there is a movement away from this surgical practice. In Europe and other parts of the world, circumcision has never been routinely performed except on members of the Jewish faith. The position of the American Academy of Pediatrics, the American College of Obstetrics and Gynecology, and the American Pediatric Urological Society is that the routine circumcision of newborns is not medically indicated. Contrary to prior belief, it has not been found to prevent cancer in later life, and it does not have a significant impact on the incidence of urinary tract infections. It is surgery with its attendant risks: The penis can be damaged, and infections from the surgery are not uncommon. There may be psychological damage as well.

During the operation, the foreskin must be torn away from the glans with a blunt probe, as these two tissues have not yet separated naturally. This tearing is not only quite painful but creates scarring and thickening over the normal mucosal surface of the glans, which results in progressive sensitivity loss that will affect the person as an adult. During sexual activity, the intact foreskin slides back off the glans and covers the shaft. This skin is loosely attached so there is freedom of motion. The erect penis of the circumcised male has none of this mobile skin: What is cut would have become one-third to one-half of the penile skin necessary to accommodate a full and comfortable erection. As a result, erections in the circumcised male may be painful; artificial lubrication may be necessary for both participants; and since many of the sensitive nerves have been removed with the foreskin, the sex act may be less than satisfactory. The foreskin also protects the head of the infant penis from diaper rash, urine, and feces.

The safest care of the uncircumcised penis is to leave it alone. If the foreskin is pulled back before the lining skin has completely formed, tearing, pain, and scar formation can result. Normal maturity and epithelization take three to ten years.

CLUMSINESS (See Crawling)

COLDS

COLDS ARE viral infections that are common in children. Symptoms may begin with fever, after which a clear discharge drains from the nose over a period of about a week, often accompanied by cough and irritability. If the discharge becomes green or yellow, a secondary bacterial infection is indicated. Estimates are that there are about one hundred different cold viruses, and children are exposed to a number of them every year. Children are starting school and day care, mixing with other children, and exposing themselves to more frequent infections at a younger age than they once did.

Children are particularly prone to colds because their immune systems are immature. Rising to the challenge of these minor ailments helps them develop strong immune systems. The coughing and sneezing that characterize the cold are the body's attempt to get rid of offending irritants. If cold symptoms are suppressed with drugs, toxins can be driven inward, where they can do long-term damage to internal organs. Colds should be regarded as beneficial cleaning processes and allowed to run their course.

 Drug Treatment

OVER $2 BILLION is spent annually in the United States on over-the-counter cough and cold remedies, although these drugs have no effect on the length of the disease. They can also produce side effects, a problem that is compounded in the popular products consisting of several ingredients in fixed combinations. Typically, the multiple drugs they contain aren't necessary, and their side effects are multiplied correspondingly.

Topical decongestants can instantly open the nasal passages. The problem is that "rebound congestion" follows two or three hours later. The nasal passages swell to worse than their original condition, and the sufferer can sleep through the night only with another dose of the drug.

Antibiotics are even more problematic. Well over a million prescriptions are written each year for antibiotics for the common cold, yet these drugs have no effect on the viruses to which colds are attributed.

The expressed justification is prophylactic—to treat any bacterial infection that *might* arise. The problems with this theory are that if an infection does develop, the bacteria will have had an opportunity to adapt to the drug, rendering it ineffective; and the patient runs the unnecessary risk of developing an allergic reaction to it.

 ## Natural Alternatives

NATUROPATHIC DOCTORS contend that cold symptoms are natural cleansing processes that should not be suppressed. Sufferers report that when they give up cold-treatment drugs, the condition becomes more tolerable of its own accord. When they refrain from decongestants, the overall course of their congestion is more manageable. Colds left to run their course get progressively milder and further apart as the body succeeds in its attempted housecleaning.

Meanwhile, natural remedies can ease cold symptoms effectively without side effects. Elderberry extract (Sambucus nigra) is a very popular herbal remedy. Rather than merely suppressing the body's eliminatory mechanisms, elderberry extract has been shown to actually halt the spread of the cold virus. A recent study suggests that it can significantly reduce the length and severity of flu symptoms.[68] An Israeli study showed an extract of the herb to cut recovery times in half.[69]

Olive-leaf extract is another herb shown in medical studies to eliminate bacteria and viruses from the body.[70]

Echinacea is a third popular herbal option. It is quite effective if used at the right stage of a cold, at the first sign of symptoms. If it is used at the wrong stage, clinical practice suggests that it can actually worsen symptoms. The Chinese explanation is that it strengthens the *wei chi,* the protective energy layer on the outside of the body that stops things from going in or out. At the first stage of a cold, echinacea prevents pathogens from getting in; but once they are in, it can trap them inside. People who complain they've been sick with a cold for several weeks

("It just won't seem to go away") frequently turn out to be taking echinacea. The herb should be taken only when the patient feels like he or she might be "coming down with something." Once the illness hits in force, it's too late. The remedy is a good one to give when your child is not sick but is around children who are. At that stage, it strengthens the body's internal energy and protects it from invasion.

Early-stage colds can often be halted in their tracks with a homeopathic product made by Dolisos called Cold and Flu Solution Plus. (Make sure the label says "Plus"; there is also a plain Cold and Flu Solution.) Use one tablet every fifteen minutes for the first hour, then one tablet every hour for the next four hours, then one tablet four times daily. Another good homeopathic option is Viral CM by CompliMed.

A third effective homeopathic approach is a combination of Alpha CF by B&T and Oscillococcinum by Boiron. Mix two tablets of Alpha CF and one tube of Oscillococcinum in an eight-ounce glass of water. Two ounces should be drunk every fifteen minutes until the water is gone. Make another mixture in water in the same proportions, to be drunk at the rate of two ounces every hour until gone.

A good diet supplemented with vitamin C and other vitamins and minerals can shorten the length and frequency of colds. Numerous studies have found that vitamin-C supplements taken at a dose of 1,000 milligrams or more daily while cold symptoms last can significantly reduce symptoms and help speed recovery. Benefits appear to be greater for children than for adults. As for taking high doses of vitamin C daily when well to prevent colds, there is no real evidence that this approach is effective unless the immune system has been weakened for some reason or a deficiency of the vitamin exists. The exact dose to use during colds is debated, but a typical recommendation is 500 to 1,000 milligrams three to six times daily while cold symptoms last. The short-term use of high doses of vitamin C is believed to be safe, although diarrhea may occur.[71] The safety of taking high doses of vitamin C long-term has been questioned, because vitamin C is an acid that can leach calcium (a buffering base) from the bones.

For children, Emer'gen-C, an effervescent vitamin C, is a great remedy at the beginning of a cold. It gets the vitamin into the system faster than tablets, and children love the fizz and variety of flavors.

Clinical studies have shown zinc gluconate to help at the first stage of a cold. Sucking on zinc lozenges can help stop an incipient cold by acting directly on the virus on the surface of the throat and tonsils.

Some physicians favor the use of old-fashioned remedies: chicken soup; mixtures of spirits, honey, and lemon juice; hot milk and honey; herbal teas. Studies have shown that hot drinks make the cold sufferer feel better by increasing the flow of nasal secretions.[72]

Licorice-root tea is good for opening the bronchioles of the chest. Use should be limited to two cups a day, however, since large amounts can cause water retention and increase blood pressure.

Colostrum, derived from the first milk of cows, is an effective immune system booster that is now available in pill form. In many reported cases, taking colostrum capsules every hour or two at the first sign of a cold has kept the cold from developing.

A cell salt called Bioplasma is another popular alternative for building immunity in kids. Cell salts are homeopathic remedies made from salts occurring naturally in the body. Bioplasma is easy to take, tastes like candy, and dissolves easily. The recommended dose is four pills three times a day. A homeopathic product called Thymactive by NF Formulas is also quite effective in boosting the immature immune systems of preschoolers and kindergartners.

For other immune system boosters, see "Immunity."

 ## Chinese Herbal Remedies

CHINESE DOCTORS use different herbal remedies for a cold, depending on its stage and symptoms. They view the first stage as being on the "outside"—the surface of the body. The symptoms are chills, aches and pains, headache, possibly a slight sore throat, stiff neck, and an aversion to cold air or wind. The cold that has progressed beyond this stage goes "inside" and turns "hot," producing fever and yellow-green sputum. It can go to the sinuses and cause a sinus infection, or to the chest and cause bronchitis. Appropriate Chinese remedies for various stages and types of colds are designated below. All Chinese formulas should be taken with warm water for best results—not mixed with water, but drunk down with it. Dosages vary with age and weight and are listed on the product packaging, but it's best to consult a qualified practitioner.

For the cold that is just beginning or for the flulike cold with nausea:

At the beginning of a cold, there is a sensation of being either hot or cold. There may be sore throat, mild fever, body aches, or headache. The appropriate remedy is Gan Mao Ling. This is also the appropriate remedy when the cold goes to nausea, severe aches, and headache.

For the second-stage cold:

When the cold has set in a little more—the patient is feeling worse and anticipates feeling quite miserable tomorrow—the appropriate Chinese formula is Yin Chiao. The dosage is three to four pills, three to four times daily, with warm water or added to boiling water as a tea.

For a cold with fever:

Zhong Gan Ling is effective for high fever (the distinguishing trait for this remedy) with sore throat or strep throat and body aches. K'an Herbs makes a version for children called Zhong Gan Ling Jr.

When the patient is coughing up yellow or green phlegm:

The Chinese maintain that this symptom indicates the cold has gone deep into the body and has gotten very hot, making the phlegm turn yellow. Constipation is often present as the body fluids are burned off. The remedy is Ching Fei Yi Huo, three pills two to three times daily.

For strep throat:

Lu-Shen-Wan, when given for a very sore throat with fever, has been known to cure the condition in a single day.

COLD SORES, CANKER SORES

COLD SORES (fever blisters) and canker sores (aphthous ulcers) are two of the most common infections of the mouth. Cold sores are most likely to appear on the outside of the mouth and lips, although they can show up anywhere on the skin or on the gums. Canker sores are small, painful ulcers on the inside of the mouth, usually lasting five to ten days. An important difference is that canker sores are not thought to be contagious, while cold sores are. Cold sores may be accompanied by fever, swollen neck glands, and a general achy feeling. Canker sores are rarely accompanied by fever or other signs of illness.

The cause of canker sores is unknown, but they may be due to allergy, nutritional deficiencies, or defects in the immune system. Stress or sensitivity to some foods (tomato, chocolate, citrus) may trigger them.

Cold sores are caused by the herpes simplex virus. Exposure to this virus is common, but infections result only when resistance is low, as from a cold, sunburn, shock, dental or sinus infection, or menstruation. Originally, there were two principal strains of herpes simplex virus, type 1 and type 2; but the strains have now crossed. Type 1, or oral herpes, is the usual cause of cold sores, but type 2, once limited to the genital region, may now also produce cold sores on the face. Touching cold sores can result in spreading the virus to new sites on the body including the genitals, or to other people, so it's important to keep hands off and avoid kissing. Once oral herpes has been contracted, the virus remains in a nerve near the cheekbone, and outbreaks can recur. As with genital herpes, oral herpes outbreaks have been linked to emotional stress, as well as to fever, illness, injury, and overexposure to sun.

Cold sores in newborns may manifest in multiple organs, the nervous system, or just the skin, eyes, or mouth. Systemic (whole-body) involvement carries a high risk of death. All pregnant women should be asked about recent genital herpes infection. For a woman ready to deliver who has active genital lesions, Cesarean delivery is suggested.

Conventional Treatment

ANTISEPTIC POWDERS and ointments may be used to prevent secondary infections, and various lotions and powders can relieve pain and itching and hasten drying; but there is no pharmaceutical cure for these skin eruptions, and the drugs used on them can have side effects. The antiviral drug acyclovir (Zovirax) may be used topically for cold sores, but the blisters tend to recur.[73] Zovirax can also have side effects, including nausea and vomiting, diarrhea, headache, and skin rash. It does not work on canker sores, for which steroids like hydrocortisone cream are typically recommended instead; but these, too, can have harmful side effects (see "Itching"), and they suppress the body's own efforts at cure.

 Natural Alternatives

COLD SORES and canker sores really need no treatment at all; but if the sores are particularly bothersome or recurring, natural remedies can relieve discomfort and speed healing.

Homeopathic Borax 6x helps to rapidly heal canker-sore blisters. The dosage is three pills, three times daily. Hydrastis MT (mother tincture) is another homeopathic remedy that soothes and heals canker sores. Dilute at the rate of one part to ten parts distilled water. Rinse with the liquid, then spit it out. Pantothenic acid may help relieve canker-sore pain. If your child is prone to canker sores, avoid serving acidic or spicy foods and any foods to which he or she may be allergic.

For cold sores, the most well-known natural alternative is the amino acid lysine. Dosage is one gram every four hours at the outset, or 500 milligrams twice or three times a day to prevent recurrences.

Lysine works, and it is safer than Zovirax; but it still addresses only the symptoms. Homeopathic remedies not only can heal cold sores but can prevent them from coming back. Homeopathic Calendula and

Hypericum Ointment by Boiron clears the blisters up quickly, while Natrum muraticum (Nat mur) 6x keeps them from recurring. The recommended dosage of Nat mur is four pills, four times daily, at the onset of symptoms. Although the cold sores may seem at first to be recurring more often but healing faster, in a few months they should be gone for good. For stubborn cases, a single dose of Herpes simplex homeopathic nosode may also be given. Other effective homeopathic options include Cold Sores by Natra-Bio and Kliniskin H by Klinica (also good for herpes).

Other natural topical remedies that aid in healing cold sores include herbal Goldenseal-Propolis Cream by Eclectic Institute, Lic-gel by Scientific Botanicals, and Erpace by Dolisos.

Recurring Cold Sores Eliminated

An eight-year-old girl was miserable with recurring cold sores, breaking out with them every couple of weeks. The homeopathic remedy Nat mur 6x succeeded in breaking this cycle when conventional treatment had failed.

COLIC

COLIC IS a period of unexplained, prolonged, inconsolable crying in an infant. The baby's loud, piercing cries typically peak in late afternoon or evening. The knees may draw up, the abdomen becomes tense, and the face turns red as if from gas and indigestion. A common cause is a sensitivity to cow's-milk formula, but colic may occur in breast-fed as well as in formula-fed babies. Another possible cause is *anal ring,* a partial obstruction just inside the anal opening. About one in four children has this temporary problem. Fortunately, babies usually outgrow the colicky phase by four months of age.

Medical Treatment

SIMETHICONE DROPS, which decrease bowel gas without getting absorbed into the system, are considered safe; but studies have not shown any real benefit for colic.[74] In the case of unremitting colic, glycerin suppositories may be recommended to help the baby expel the gas or feces that may be causing his discomfort. Other drugs, including antiflatulents, sedatives, and antispasmodics such as dicyclomine (Bentyl), are sometimes prescribed for colic and occasionally offer limited relief, but in most cases they are of little benefit, and they can have harmful side effects.[75]

If colic is caused by anal ring, the insertion of a lubricated little finger or a suppository may both diagnose and treat the problem. This procedure needs to be performed by a doctor.

 ## Home Care

FIRST RULE out hunger. Parents may feel their baby could not be hungry after only two hours has elapsed since the last feeding, but a baby's stomach can actually empty in an hour, so try a feeding if that time has passed. Babies need about two ounces of food per pound per day. That means an eight-pound baby should be getting at least sixteen ounces of food. Growth is so fast in infancy that if it were to continue at the same rate throughout life as in the first two weeks, the child would be twenty-two feet tall by the time he was ten years old. That rate of growth requires constant feeding. Many women just carry their babies around with them all day and let feeding occur at will. If fed every two hours during the day, an infant may actually sleep for six to eight hours at night.

If colic is due to milk sensitivity, milk alternatives can help. Try soy milk, goat's milk, or meat-based formulas. (See "Nutrition.")

Chinese medicine considers "cold in the stomach" to be the cause of colic, either from drinking cold milk or formula or from being left with the stomach uncovered. The solution is to warm the baby's stomach with a tea made from fennel seed given at room temperature. Another alternative is Grippe Water, popular in England and in Armenian grocery stores.

An effective homeopathic remedy for colic is Cocyntal by Boiron. It comes in a water base and can be given every three hours as needed. Alpha TLC is another homeopathic remedy for colic that comes in tablet form.

Rescue Remedy, a Bach flower remedy, is an excellent option for assuaging tears and discomfort.

Some Creative Solutions to Challenging Colic Cases

Some babies seem to be sensitive to every feeding alternative. One infant got a rash with cow's milk, got colic with soy milk, got diarrhea with goat's milk, and spit up much of a meat-based formula. The compromise solution: The mother used cow's milk on Monday, soy milk on Tuesday, goat's milk on Wednesday, and meat-based formula on Thursday. Another baby was sensitive to all of these alternatives. Simmering skim milk for five hours was found to denature the milk enough that, while the infant still had runny green stools, he held the milk down and cried less.

Another mother found that her infant's "colic" was really a broken collarbone, suffered when this large baby was squeezed through the birth canal. The key to diagnosis was that he cried when picked up. He healed easily in just a few weeks.

A mother who had tried everything to stop her baby's crying and was at her wit's end delightedly reported that a single dose of Rescue Remedy stopped the infant's tears immediately.

While you are waiting for the colicky phase to pass, hold the baby rather than letting him or her cry alone. Positions that put natural pressure against the abdomen can help. Try sitting in a comfortable chair and placing the baby facedown, stomach across your knees, Another option is to hold the baby on your forearm, with the baby's stomach along your arm and the head at the crook of your elbow, holding the baby's body securely by the leg near the diaper. Slow rocking is better than bouncing or jiggling. Just the gentle pressure of your warm body against the baby's stomach works for many infants. You can also massage the abdomen by placing your hands at the bottom of the baby's rib cage, then gently and slowly moving them, palms downward, to the thighs. When the crying gets to be too much, leave your baby with a relative or baby-sitter and take a break—an option that will help both of you!

CONCUSSION (See Head Injury)

CONJUNCTIVITIS (See Eye Infection)

CONSTIPATION

CONSTIPATION IS the passage of infrequent, hard, dry stools. It is defined as an irregular retention or delay in bowel movements, but "irregular" is a relative term. More important than frequency is the consistency of the stools. Breast-fed babies often pass them only every few days, but the stools are soft and easy to pass. Babies fed on cow's milk often have large, hard bowel movements. These babies need some roughage.

Constipation can also be triggered by certain drugs. Common offenders include codeine, antihistamines, diuretics, antispasmodics, narcotics, sleeping pills, antidepressants, tranquilizers, and iron supplements.

Pharmaceutical Treatment

AVOID USE of laxative drugs. Laxatives diminish the natural muscle reflexes, so peristalsis occurs only with stronger and stronger stimulation. The drugs can also irritate and inflame the lining of the bowel, cause anal fissures and hemorrhoids, and deplete the body of important substances, including water, calcium, potassium, and magnesium. The safest drugstore constipation remedies are the bulk-forming and stool-softening varieties that encourage normal bowel function. The bulk-formers (like Metamucil) generally contain psyllium seed, while the stool softeners (like Doxidan) generally contain docusate.

Natural Solutions

MOST IMPORTANT is to change the diet from low-fiber to high-fiber. Fiber helps soften and increase the weight of stools, prevent straining, and speed intestinal transit time. Wheat bran is often recommended, but pure wheat bran can irritate the delicate lining of the intestines and inhibit mineral absorption. The same laxative effect can be achieved with whole foods containing fiber. Raw vegetables, raw and dried fruits, and most beans and whole grains are high in it. They create a heavy intestinal mass that travels quickly through the intestines. Reduce or avoid foods devoid of fiber: That means animal foods, especially cheese, and refined foods, especially sugar.

Proper toilet training and toilet habits are also important. A child needs to learn to avoid haste, to allow time for nature to take its course, and to respond when it calls. Sufficient water drinking is also important. (See "Nutrition.")

Beneficial bacteria (acidophilus and bifidus) can aid elimination. They are found in yogurt but can be obtained in much greater quantity if taken in capsule or liquid form. PB-8 by Nutrition Now is particularly good for kids. It contains eight different types of acidophilus in powdered form. The same company also makes flavored chewable aci-dophilus tablets.

Greens and green-type nutritional supplements can help clean the liver, add fiber, and facilitate bowel movements. Green supplements include chlorella, spirulina, and blue-green algae. Taking spirulina or chlorella twice a day typically results in normal bowel movements in about four days.

Aloe vera juice taken orally can also help; a brand called George's is particularly good. It may be taken alone or with juice in the morning, in a dosage varying with age and ranging from one teaspoon to two table-spoons.

Wineberry is a gemmotherapy useful in the treatment of constipation.

Homeopathic remedies can help chronic constipation. BHI makes a good homeopathic combination called Constipation. For addressing the emotional element ("holding things in"), Nat mur is very effective.

Traumatized Boy's Constipation Relieved Homeopathically

A young boy who was routinely being picked on by his more aggressive twin brother was chronically constipated. His parents had tried enemas, but they only traumatized him further. A course of Nat mur along with increased water-drinking resolved his consti-pation completely.

CONVULSIONS (See Seizures)

COUGHS

A COUGH is a protective reflex for eliminating foreign substances that block the airways. There are two types of cough, wet and dry. Wet coughs are productive: They are bringing something up. Dry coughs are unproductive and are liable to be a sign of sinus problems. Although coughs go with colds, they can last long after the cold is gone. Other conditions for which coughs may be a symptom include postnasal drip, allergies, sinus infection, and asthma. Coughs with high fever, wheezing, pressure in the head, dizziness, or painful teeth should be checked by a qualified practitioner.

 ## Drug Treatment

THE FDA warns that drugs that suppress the protective cough reflex can do more harm than good. Cough suppressants are recommended only for dry coughs. They aren't recommended for people with asthma and other conditions involving overproduction of secretions, since these coughs, while chronic and annoying, are still productive. That means most coughs are best left alone.

 ## Natural Alternatives

COUGH & BRONCHIAL Syrup by B&T, Cough Solution by Dolisos, and Cough by Natra-Bio are effective natural cough remedies. Herbs for Kids makes a Cherry Bark Blend cough formula that is alcohol-free. Chestal by Boiron is another popular natural cough remedy, but it should not be used by children less than one year old because it contains honey, which poses a remote risk of botulism. (See "Nutrition.")

Aromatherapy, involving the essential oils of plants, can also help alleviate cough symptoms. Try rubbing the chest with essential oil of eucalyptus or myrrh.

Another way to loosen a child's nasal secretions is to have him breathe the steam from a vaporizer or hot shower, or use mustard plasters. (For directions, see "Bronchitis.")

For other natural cough remedies that work, see "Colds."

CRADLE CAP

CRADLE CAP is a form of seborrhea—an excessive secretion of the sebaceous glands of the skin—manifesting as yellow, greasy scales on the head of an infant. Because cradle cap provides a fertile ground for the growth of bacteria and fungi, a secondary bacterial infection frequently contaminates the weepy rawness behind the ears.

 Natural Remedies

CRADLE CAP can be controlled by rubbing a few drops of a natural oil into the affected area. Herbs for Kids makes a Cradle Cap Oil that is good. Another option is flaxseed oil. The scales on the head may then come off in the bath. Soap and a soft brush can help remove extra scales. Mothers sometimes worry about touching the "soft spot" at the top of the head, but the tissues there are tough, so one needn't worry about accidentally damaging the brain. To avoid secondary fungal infections, dry the baby's armpits and between the fingers and toes thoroughly. Try cornstarch on those areas. Perfumed oils can provoke sensitivity reactions and are not necessary; nonallergenic oils or creams are the best products to use on scaly skin.

Colloidal silver is a relatively old solution for cradle cap that is making a comeback. It has germicidal properties and can be painted on the affected area with a cotton swab. Within two to three days, the cradle cap should dissolve.

For candida infection or secondary bacterial infection, first try a bland cream like Calendula or Herbs for Kids' Cradle Cap Oil. If redness remains, the conventional solution is a cortisone ointment, but homeopaths maintain that this merely pushes the infection deeper into the system. A solution of homeopathic Candida taken orally is a safer alternative.

One possible cause of cradle cap is vitamin B_6 deficiency. If the mother experienced nausea and vomiting during pregnancy and has trouble with dream recall, she may be lacking in that vitamin and may have passed the deficiency to her baby. In those cases, supplementing the baby's diet with vitamin B_6 may help.

CRAMPS (See Menstrual Problems)

CRAWLING, DEVELOPMENTAL LAGS, ACCIDENT-PRONENESS

AWKWARDNESS AND accident-proneness may have a physical cause such as anoxia (lack of oxygen, usually occurring at the time of delivery) or other injury to the nervous system. However, these traits are also commonly seen in hyperactive children whose actions are simply ahead of their coordination. The awkward child may just be experiencing a developmental lag. (See also "Dyslexia.")

 Natural Therapy

FLORENCE SCOTT, R.N., a neurodevelopmental specialist in Woodburn, Oregon, has derived a form of neurodevelopmental therapy called patterning, which uses the stimulation of creeping (moving like a lizard) and crawling (moving on hands and knees). If a child or adult has had an injury to the nervous system from infection or trauma, this method of therapy can help reattach the "breaks" in the nervous system. Neurodevelopmental stimulation from crawling and creeping is an important step in maturity. The floor is the infant's gym. Crawling is the infant's first means of locomotion and usually occurs at about three to six months of age. The slithering movements not only help the baby program the right/left aspects of his world but have been found to be important preparations for reading. The messages from the arms and legs imprint on the cortex of the brain in preparation for later academic functions. It has been documented that babies who were placed in walkers in infancy have more trouble learning to read, evidently because they do not get the stimulation afforded by crawling and creeping. Walkers are also hazardous for mechanical reasons, including their tendency to roll down stairs and should not be used. For further information, call Florence Scott at 503-981-0635 or e-mail nntc@open.org.

CROSSED EYES (See Visual Problems)

CROUP, EPIGLOTTITIS (VOCAL-CORD INFLAMMATION)

CROUP IS an inflammation of the larynx that causes the child to produce a characteristic barking sound. The condition usually manifests in the middle of the night after a warm, dry day followed by a cool, dry night. At about midnight the parents are awakened by what they think is a barking dog or seal in the nursery. Croup is a mild inflammation that lasts about three days and involves no fever, distinguishing it from the more serious epiglottitis.

Epiglottitis is an inflammation of the area just beneath the vocal cords caused by bacterial infection. The child wakens with a dry, barking cough and high fever, and the chest heaves with each breath. The condition can be very serious or fatal, as the child becomes exhausted fighting for breath. The lips and face may go blue. Unlike simple croup, which is usually calmed with steam alone, epiglottitis barely responds to steam. When croup is present with fever, call the doctor immediately.

 ## Conventional Treatment

THE PEDIATRICIAN will prescribe antibiotics for epiglottitis, and hospitalization may be required. Serious cases may need surgical treatment, which involves making a hole in the trachea below the obstruction so that breathing is easier. Oxygen is also routinely given in the hospital.

For croup, the treatment conventionally recommended is antibiotics and steroids.[76] For downsides, see "Immunity."

 ## Home Treatment

FOR CROUP, hold the child upright and have her swallow some lemon or other juice mixed with honey. Gin, lemon juice, and honey is an old-time favorite. (Children under one year old should not have honey—see "Nutrition." Parents can decide about the gin.) Keep the room warm and humid, and give steam inhalation if possible. Use a humidifier, or have the child stand in the bathroom with the shower running hot enough to fog up the mirror, or hang wet sheets and towels around the bedroom. This should calm her enough to make sleep possible. If the child cannot relax and sleep, if difficulty in breathing persists, or if there is a fever, seek medical attention.

Homeopathic remedies are also available. For croup, give Rumex (for a barking, seal-like cough). Aconite (for any illness of sudden onset) may also be given every fifteen minutes for two hours or until the fever goes down; then give Spongia every two hours until you see improvement. For cases involving abundant phlegm in the lungs, give the homeopathic remedy Antim tart. If you hear rattling in the chest, give Hepar sulph.

For epiglottitis, call the doctor immediately if there is fever; but homeopathic remedies may be given to ease symptoms. If the child feels hot and is restless, give Belladonna 30c or 200c (whichever is available), three tablets every few hours. At the early onset of symptoms, use Bacticin by CompliMed, ten drops three times daily. If the child has swollen glands, use Inflammation by CompliMed, ten drops three times daily.

Croup Cured with Homeopathic Remedies

A three-year-old boy with a dry, barking cough was given homeopathic Rumex. Within a few hours, the cough made a more normal sound of mucus in the chest. The remedy was then changed to Antim tart. The amazed mother reported that after two doses, the croup was gone and the boy was well.

CUTS (see Abrasions)

CYSTIC FIBROSIS

CYSTIC FIBROSIS is a hereditary disease in which children produce insufficient digestive enzymes. Symptoms include foul-smelling stools and chronic bronchitis. Chronic lung congestion then produces pressure on the right side of the heart. The condition is so serious that these children rarely survive to young adulthood.

Drug Treatment

ANTIBIOTICS ARE often prescribed for the bronchial inflammation characterizing cystic fibrosis, but the drugs will not reverse its fatal course.

Natural Alternatives

RECENT RESEARCH indicates that pancreatic enzymes and selenium can help control the symptoms of cystic fibrosis.[77]

CYSTITIS (See Bladder Infection)

DEAFNESS (See Hearing Impairment)

DENTAL PROBLEMS: TOOTHACHE, TOOTH DECAY, TOOTHBRUSHING, TEETHING, MALOCCLUSION, TMJ (Temporomandibular Joint) DYSFUNCTION, TOOTH INJURIES, TOOTH GRINDING

TOOTHACHE CAN have a variety of causes, including tooth decay, teething, and a misaligned bite.

Tooth decay or *dental caries* occur in the enamel and dentin of the teeth, when acid formed by bacteria feeding on retained food particles (especially sugar) create holes in the enamel and eventually the pulp. Infants allowed to fall asleep with bottles propped in their mouths are liable to develop rampant caries unless the bottle contains only water. Poor toothbrushing, sticky candies, and a deficiency of magnesium in the diet all tend to increase the incidence of tooth decay. Breast milk has a high content of magnesium, and so do most vegetables.

The baby's teeth should be brushed from the time they start coming in at about six months of age. Parents should continue this project for several years, until children can be trusted to do it themselves. Baby or primary teeth will be shed, but if they contain caries, they should be treated by a dentist, as infected pulp may lead to abscesses and complications. A dental abscess (an infection in the tissue surrounding the tooth root) can jeopardize the health of the entire body.

Teething may make infants irritable when the teeth are pushing painfully through the gums. The first molars come after the central and lateral incisors. The cuspids fill in the space between the incisors and the molars by about eighteen months. The second molars usually come all at once by about age two. If the first permanent lower incisors have not erupted by age seven, an X ray may be prudent to see if they are there. Occasionally low thyroid function will explain the delay. Besides gum pain, teething may be responsible for a range of apparently unrelated conditions, including stomachaches, sugar cravings, irritability, bad behavior, headaches, and sleeplessness. Because the meridians, or energy systems, that run through the mouth go through almost every vital organ, teething can disrupt the whole body.

A condition related to teething is the appearance of a blue-eruption hematoma (a cyst of blood) between the crown of a molar and the unbroken gum. It is rarely necessary to cut the gums in these cases, since the growth force of the tooth is stronger than the gum tissue through which it is emerging. The tooth will erupt of its own accord.

Crowding of primary teeth is obvious by age four. Babies who have been breast-fed for a year or so rarely have crowded teeth. (See "Breast-feeding.")

Malocclusion, or the inability of the teeth to make even contact when the jaws bite together, may involve an overbite or an underbite. An overbite may be caused by the use of bottled formula in infancy, or by thumb sucking. However, thumb sucking does not seem to be harmful to the teeth until the permanent teeth erupt, when it should be discouraged. (See "Nail Biting.")

Temporomandibular joint (TMJ) dysfunction is pain arising in the jaw joint. It can result from a faulty bite. When the bite is off, so is the TMJ, which has an energetic relationship with areas all over the body. X rays have verified that when missing or short back teeth cause the bite to overclose, the many nerves that originate in the neck get pinched through the cervical plexus. Neurological symptoms follow, including pain, headaches, backaches, and fatigue. Harold Gelb, D.M.D., a professor of dentistry and founder of the Gelb Craniomandibular and Orofacial Pain Center at Tufts University School of Dental Medicine, lists a host of other seemingly unrelated symptoms, including chronic sore throat, asthma, upset stomach, diarrhea, arthritis, lowered thyroid activity, depression, and forgetfulness.[78]

Displacement of baby teeth and injuries to them should be evaluated by a dentist. Some teeth need to be replaced or held in place to maintain the space for the permanent teeth. An avulsed tooth—one that comes out root and all—can sometimes be replaced in the socket and saved, but this must be done within about thirty minutes of the injury for the tooth to reattach.

Tooth grinding is generally considered a sign of tension. However, nighttime grinding can also be a symptom of pinworms. (See "Parasites.")

 ## Conventional Treatment: Fluoride, Mercury Amalgam, and Other Dental Controversies

FLUORIDE IS the conventional solution to the problem of tooth decay, but whether its benefits outweigh its burdens is controversial. In a series of studies comparing cancer death rates in fluoridated and unfluoridated populations, fluoridated cities showed an approximate 10 percent increase in cancer deaths. The researchers concluded from this and other evidence that fluoridation may account for more than thirty thousand deaths a year in the United States, of which more than ten thousand are due to cancer. To make matters worse, the researchers demonstrated that adding fluoride to the water supply has *no* significant impact on dental caries.[79] A 1986–87 oral health survey involving 39,207 U.S. schoolchildren found a continuing decline in caries prevalence in both fluoridated and unfluoridated areas, leading the researchers to conclude that "caries is no longer a public health problem."[80]

Other dental controversies include the use of silver/mercury for filling caries and gutta-percha for filling root canals. These materials have now been linked to a host of long-term chronic ailments. For a fuller discussion, and for some recent refinements in children's dental care that can make dental visits painless, see Ellen Brown and Richard Hansen, D.M.D., *The Key to Ultimate Health*.[81]

Natural Alternatives for Avoiding Caries

RESEARCH HAS shown that many "primitive" people around the world have teeth that are free of cavities, gum disease, and orthodontic defects, although they do not have the benefit of dentists, orthodontists, fluoride, or even toothbrushes.[82] In the forties, Harold Hawkins, D.D.S., showed that if the mineral levels of the saliva were raised to sufficient levels, cavities would be totally eliminated. This was true for children who never used fluoride or even brushed their teeth.[83] In the same decade, Weston Price, D.D.S., documented cases of spontaneous regeneration of teeth that originally were so decayed that the inner pulp was exposed. After the children's nutrition was improved, the teeth reincased themselves in secondary dentin (the tooth tissue under the hard outer enamel), drawing on the minerals in the saliva to rebuild themselves.[84]

A little-recognized factor in tooth health is proper lighting. Research has shown that people exposed to full-spectrum fluorescent light (visible and UV) have substantially fewer dental caries than those exposed to conventional fluorescent light.[85] Besides sunshine, full-spectrum lighting may be obtained from special lightbulbs available in health food stores.

 ## Natural Alternatives for Relieving Dental Pain

HOMEOPATHIC AND herbal remedies can help relieve teething and dental pain. The usual homeopathic remedy for teething is Chamomile. Herbs for Kids makes a Gum-omile Oil Blend Liquid for teething and other dental pain. Rescue Remedy, a Bach flower remedy, applied directly to the gums can relax the baby, decrease stress, and relieve pain. Chewing on a pacifier or rubber ring may be soothing to the gums. Homeopathic remedies can also speed the eruption of teeth.

Give Calc carb 200x (three pills three times in one day, then stop), or Calc phos 6x (three pills two times daily for one week).

Effective homeopathic remedies for dental pain include Gunpowder 6x (three pills four times daily) and Bacticin (ten drops every hour). Pyrogenium (two every couple of hours as needed) expels pus. If pus or a bad taste appears in the mouth, don't panic; it means the remedy is working. For dental pain from inflammation, Hypericum 30c is reported to work as well as aspirin without its side effects (excess bleeding, stomach upset, nausea). Take three pills four times daily.

For relief from the swelling and pain of dental abscess, a German Staufen homeopathic remedy called Corynebacterium Anaerobius Nosode is excellent. In the United States, Deseret makes a dental formula that contains this nosode.

Herbal remedies for temporary relief from toothache include oil of clove applied directly to the painful tooth. Another home remedy reported to work is to apply a few drops of a liquid extract of echinacea and goldenseal directly to the tooth. Leave for a few hours or overnight, freshening periodically.

Symptoms of TMJ dysfunction have been relieved by correcting the bite, either with Gelb-type acrylic splints or with orthodontia. TMJ problems may be caused in the newborn by a tumultuous delivery or in older children by simple tension. For the latter, consciously relaxing the TMJ muscle can realign the jaw. A homeopathic remedy called TMJ by New Vista can help relieve symptoms. Chiropractic or craniosacral adjustment may also help. Cranial therapy can help preclude later orthodontic care, spreading the palate without loss of teeth.

Stomachaches Relieved with Teething Remedy

Danielle, age seven, had chronic stomach problems. Her mother was in despair, as no cause or cure could be found. Testing linked the problem to the girl's teeth. She was given Chamomile, the homeopathic remedy for teething, and all her stomach problems disappeared.

DEPRESSION

AN ESTIMATED fifteen million American adults and children are clinically depressed. Adolescents are the most likely preadult group, but the condition can also strike younger children. Depression is a state of deep sadness, irritablity, boredom, and hopelessness. While it is natural after a death or other serious loss or disappointment, time should heal the wound. When depression lasts more than two weeks or interferes with normal activities, additional help may be required. Besides lowered mood, symptoms of depression can include feelings of guilt, worthlessness, or hopelessness; loss of energy or appetite; insufficient or excessive sleep; bed-wetting in young children; destructive or aggressive behavior; a drop in school performance; and withdrawal from family and friends. Teenagers may abuse alcohol and drugs or threaten suicide. Related ailments include bipolar disorder (alternating "up" and "down" phases formerly called manic-depression) and seasonal affective disorder or SAD (caused by too little sunlight in winter months).

Clinical depression is attributed to genetics, developmental problems, or psychosocial factors, but for many cases there is no clinically understood cause. Before a psychiatric label is imposed, physical and dietary factors should be ruled out, including anemias, food sensitivities, lack of magnesium in the diet, low thyroid function, and chronic infection.

Conventional Treatment

THE USUAL treatment for childhood depression is psychotherapy for the child and/or the family. The therapist may also prescribe antidepressant drugs, but their effectiveness on children and teenagers has not been proven.[86]

Amphetamines have been used for fifty years to give the depressed a "lift," but controlled trials have failed to establish that the drugs relieve depression significantly better than placebos.[87] The amphetamine ritalin is prescribed now for children with depression as well as for those with ADD. (See "ADD.")

Other drugs that are now being prescribed not only for adults but for children are those in a new line of antidepressants called selective serotonin reuptake inhibitors (SSRIs), including Prozac (fluoxetine), Zoloft, Paxil, and Effexor. Serotonin is a mood-elevating neurotransmitter, a natural upper that mediates depression. Serotonin inhibitors don't actually produce serotonin but are serotonin enhancers that act by inhibiting the reuptake of serotonin by the neurons, a natural process. Besides depression, these drugs are used to treat anxiety, addiction, bulimia, obesity, and a host of other ills. Common side effects of Prozac include sleeplessness, nervousness, nausea, and—ironically—anxiety and depression. Prozac has been implicated in more than a hundred civil suits and a number of criminal suits involving allegations that it caused violent behavior including murder and suicide.[88] (See "Anxiety.")

Caution: If prescription antianxiety or insomnia drugs are already being used, discontinue or switch remedies only under professional supervision.

 ## Natural Alternatives

THE NATURAL, balanced way to increase levels of serotonin is with its natural precursors, the amino acids L-tryptophan and L-tyrosine.

Tryptophan is the most effective serotonin producer currently known. It was used as a safe and natural alternative to pharmaceutical tranquilizers for nearly half a century, until it was removed from the market by the FDA in 1989 following reports of some serious side effects and deaths from its use. However, the problem was ultimately traced to contamination in a manufacturing process involving genetic engineering used by a particular Japanese manufacturer.[89] For children, safe sources of this amino acid are milk (breast or cow), pumpkin seeds, and turkey.

New on the market is a highly effective homeopathic serotonin enhancer called Serotonin by Deseret. It stimulates the body to produce its own serotonin and, like all homeopathics, is entirely safe. (See Introduction.) Many people have succeeded in weaning themselves off Prozac and emerging from their inexplicable depressions using this simple and inexpensive remedy. The dosage for young people is ten drops three times daily. Homeopathic Serotonin & Tryptophan by CompliMed is good for children who suffer from seasonal depression or from depression caused by insomnia.

The body's serotonin levels may also be raised by changing the diet. High-carbohydrate foods have been found to relieve depression, anger, tension, tiredness, and moodiness, apparently because they elevate serotonin levels.[90] Avoid sugary foods, however, since they can wreak havoc on the blood sugar level, and erratic drops in blood sugar can cause both depression and bingeing. The best carbohydrates are whole grains—oatmeal and other whole grain cereals, whole grain breads, rice, and potatoes. Exercise has also been shown to increase brain concentrations of serotonin and norepinephrine.[91] Running is well known for the "runner's high."

In the herbal line, a St.-John's-wort blend by Herbs for Kids is available for children. St.-John's-wort is the market favorite among natural remedies for depression. A review of twenty-three controlled studies published in the *British Medical Journal* in August 1997 concluded that St.-John's-wort worked as well as prescription drugs and nearly three times better than a placebo in countering depression, without the unwanted side effects accompanying drugs. Mild, reversible side effects did occur in some patients, but they were far less frequent or serious than those of pharmaceutical antidepressants.[92]

Herbs for Kids also makes a combination herbal formula for nervous and anxious children called Valerian Super Calm, along with a product called Valerian Certified Organic Drops.

Another herbal remedy for depression is Skullcap Oats by Eclectic Institute.

Rescue Remedy and other Bach flower remedies can help relieve depression and anxiety, and they are entirely safe.

Nutritional supplements can also help. One is magnesium, a mineral in which people with depression tend to be low; low magnesium levels heighten the nerve impulses that lead to nervous conditions. B vitamins can give the spirits a lift as well. For adrenal stress, try Bragg Liquid Aminos, a tasty supplement used as a condiment on food. Inositol (a cousin of glucose) and phosphatidylserine may also relieve symptoms.[93]

A recent study on bipolar disorder found that patients who did not respond to treatment with the standard drug lithium responded to treatment with choline (a vitamin of the B complex).[94]

Homeopathic Lithium (something quite different from the drug lithium) is also good for depression.

Aurum metallicum is a homeopathic remedy effective on suicidal depression.

For SAD, full-spectrum lights or blue light, customized colored glasses, and homeopathic Melatonin 12x can give relief.

 ## The Oriental Approach

IN CHINESE medicine, depression is attributed to liver stagnation. When the liver energy gets sluggish, the body becomes sluggish, and the emotions become dulled, subdued, and irritated. In children, liver stagnation can result from either dietary or emotional factors: eating a diet of junk food or suppressing anger.

The Chinese herbal formula for liver stagnation is called Hsiao Yao Wan. It stimulates the liver energy to work more actively, relieving the stagnant feeling. Depression typically lifts within a few days. American-made versions go by the brand names Relaxed Wanderer and Bupleurum & Peony. K'an Herbs makes Chinese herbal formulas for kids.

Chinese doctors also move the liver energy with greens. Chlorophyll and milk thistle are good for this purpose. An excellent product called Ultimate Green by Nature's Secret includes chlorella, blue-green algae, barley grass, wheat grass, spinach, alfalfa, kale, and turnip greens. For the Liver Cleanse Diet, see "Environmental Illness."

If depression is also linked to anxiety, palpitations, nightmares, or panic attacks, Chinese doctors say the heart meridian (the energetic line dominated by the heart) is likely to be involved. For a child over twelve with a heart meridian that is out of balance, appropriate Chinese herbal formulas are Anmien Pien, Pai Tzu Yang Hsin Wan, and Hu Po Yang Xin Dan.

DERMATITIS, ECZEMA, PSORIASIS, SCARS, DRY SKIN

DERMATITIS, OR skin inflammation, is a term that includes a range of skin conditions characterized by dry, red, itchy skin. *Eczema* is chronically itchy, inflamed skin that may be linked to allergies, asthma, stress, or heredity. *Psoriasis* is an unsightly and baffling skin disorder in which skin cells multiply much faster than normal, producing raised, white-scaled patches. Other common skin problems include scars and dry skin.

Conventional Treatment

FOR SERIOUS skin conditions such as psoriasis, corticosteroids are sometimes prescribed, but these drugs suppress the immune system and can allow the condition to spread. The psoriasis later comes back in a new location or covers a much larger area of skin, and if hydrocortisone cream is again used, the problem worsens. Homeopaths suggest the same syndrome could explain a link observed between eczema and asthma. Topical steroids prevent toxins from being excreted through the skin, but the toxins are still in the body. They are pushed deeper into the system, where they attack the lungs, causing asthma.

For minor skin problems, various drugstore topical remedies are available, but these, too, require caution, since many contain hazardous chemicals. We tend to think of drugs applied to the skin as being relatively harmless, since they're not taken into the body like those that are swallowed, but this is a misconception. Painkillers have actually been found to produce adverse reactions more frequently when applied to the skin than when swallowed. Oral drugs go through the normal detoxification processes for which the stomach, kidneys, and liver were designed. Drugs applied to the skin go directly into the bloodstream without metabolic intervention. Since babies' skin is particularly absorbent, topical painkillers should not be used on children under two without a doctor's advice. Adults and children who are allergic to foods or other substances should also be careful with these drugs.[95]

 ## The Natural Approach

MANY TOPICAL ointments are available for dry, itchy skin that are made from natural, nontoxic components. Squalane, made from shark-liver oil, softens the skin and is very good for psoriasis. Kukui Nut Oil from Hawaii is another good option.

A gemmotherapy called Cedar of Lebanon is particularly good for dry eczema. Another called Rye Grain is good for psoriasis.

Diet is important for the skin. Essential fatty acids are in short supply in the normal American diet and may need to be supplemented. Omega-3 fatty acids help build more efficient cell membranes that exclude allergy-provoking proteins. Evening primrose oil, fish oil, and essential fatty acids may be taken orally. Child Life makes a product called Essential Fatty Acids in liquid form that is easy for kids to take. Shark-liver oil can be applied directly to the skin.

For cracks and splits in the fingers during winter, try homeopathic Petroleum 6x, two pills orally two to three times daily.

For cracks in the heels, use Lycopodium 6x, two pills orally three times daily.

Green tea not only fights viral and bacterial infections but can be applied topically to prevent or reverse sun and other damage to the skin.[96]

For scars, a remedy called ScarGo by Home Health has produced dramatic results, causing scars to disappear.

 ### Tracking the Cause

FOR CHRONIC skin conditions, the underlying cause needs to be found. Often, it turns out to be food allergies. The nightshades—tomatoes, potatoes, green peppers, eggplant, hot pepper—are frequently related to skin rashes. Nightshade allergy shows as a characteristic patchy skin rash with red raised lines that look as if the child has been scratched. Parents are liable to insist their child never eats nightshades, until questioned about pizza, spaghetti, french fries, and other popular foods made with tomatoes, potatoes, or peppers. Discontinue nightshade-laden foods, then give a desensitizing homeopathic remedy that allows the child to eat nightshades occasionally without breaking out in a rash. Molecular Biologicals makes a remedy called Nightshades Antigen. Futureplex makes one called Nightshades.

Rashes Traced to Nightshades and Eliminated

A three-and-a-half-year-old girl had rashlike sores all over her body. When questioned about nightshade intake, the mother said her daughter never ate those vegetables, but further questioning revealed that the girl's diet consisted principally of pizza and SpaghettiOs. The mother tried omitting these foods from her daughter's diet, but the girl still had a rash. Then the mother learned that a neighbor was giving away huge beefsteak tomatoes, which the girl loved. When the tomatoes were discontinued, the rash went away. No remedy was needed except dietary change.

The case of Zach, fourteen, was more difficult. His body was covered with small itchy bumps that he would scratch until they bled. They had been diagnosed by an M.D. as psoriasis. When his mother was asked about Zach's intake of nightshades, she, too, said, "He never eats any of that." But further questioning revealed that he loved pizza and spaghetti and often ate potato chips. When he stopped eating those foods, he improved, but not dramatically. He was then given a homeopathic remedy called Nightshades Antigen by Molecular Biologicals (ten drops three times daily). He also took shark oil orally (as capsules three times daily) and topically (applied once or twice daily). Within a month, the improvement in his skin was much more noticeable. Although he admitted to still having a pizza "now and again," the itching and scratching stopped, and the dry patches cleared.

DEVELOPMENTAL LAGS (See Crawling)

DIABETES

Diabetes mellitus is an inherited disease in which glucose is poorly metabolized or stored. Diabetes results from insufficient production of or an inability to make use of insulin, the hormone that helps sugar get into the tissues. When the amount of glucose in the blood rises to a critical level, it appears in the urine, producing excessive loss of water and dehydration. Without enough glucose to convert to energy, the body burns fat and protein, leading to weight loss and acidosis (an imbalance in the body's acid levels). Prolonged elevated blood sugar is a risk factor for developing chronic complications such as vision loss, kidney failure, high blood pressure, cardiovascular disease, and neurological disorders.

Diabetes mellitus was once rare in childhood, but the incidence of child-onset, or type 1, diabetes is growing. Sixteen million Americans, or about 15 percent of the population, are diabetic; but 90 to 95 percent of them have type II or noninsulin-dependent diabetes (NIDDM), which shows up only in adulthood and is linked to obesity and faulty eating habits. The other 5 to 10 percent have the more serious child-onset or insulin-dependent diabetes (IDDM). In IDDM, little or no natural insulin is available for use by the body, requiring that the hormone be obtained by artificial means. Juvenile diabetes usually has a rapid, dramatic onset with excessive thirst, weakness, and coma. The affected child has multiple infections, loses weight suddenly, urinates frequently, and can slip into acidosis, which can be very serious or fatal. Other early warning signs include excessive hunger, fatigue, nausea, vomiting, blurred vision, and numbness in the extremities.

 Tracking the Cause

Genetic susceptibility is an important causative factor, but environmental factors also play a role. IDDM is an autoimmune disease that results when confused antibodies mistake the beta cells in the pancreas for foreign invaders and destroy them.[97] The overt disease may be precipitated by infection, stress, or rapid growth.

Early feeding of certain foods has been suspected of triggering diabetes, including cow's milk, wheat, and soy.[98] The known effects of wheat in celiac disease, a digestive disorder, prove that food can induce autoimmunity. (See "Celiac Disease.") The infant intestine isn't mature enough to properly digest many foods. Because large proteins can't be broken down properly, the walls of the intestines let large chunks pass into the bloodstream. The body evidently sees these extra-large proteins as foreign objects and creates antibodies to attack them as if they were invading bacteria.

Several studies have found that children newly diagnosed with type 1 diabetes tend to have elevated levels of antibodies to bovine serum albumin (BSA), a milk protein. A study reported in 1992 found that of 142 diabetic Finnish children studied, 100 percent had abnormally high levels of antibodies to BSA. These antibodies destroy the ability of the pancreas to produce insulin. Infants fed cow's milk during their first three months of life have been found to be 1.4 times more likely to develop diabetes.[99] To avoid an autoimmune reaction to cow's-milk protein, many doctors recommend breast-feeding during the first six months of life. For older children, however, the risk of cow's-milk-associated diabetes is thought to be slim. If you choose to keep an older child off milk, don't neglect to provide other sources of calcium. (See "Nutrition.")

Other foreign substances suspected of triggering diabetes are those injected into infants as vaccines. In September 2000, Dr. J. Bart Classen, M.D., an immunologist in Baltimore, Maryland, presented data suggesting that vaccines may be the largest single cause of type 1 diabetes. A causal relationship was suggested with many different vaccines, including pertussis, mumps, rubella, hepatitis B, and hemophilus influenza. The data indicated that people with vaccine-induced diabetes may not develop the disease until four or more years after receiving vaccines.[100] Researchers writing in *The Archives of Diseases in Childhood* in November 1997 also pointed to childhood immunizations as a possible cause of both diabetes and allergies.[101] For further discussion, see "Allergies."

Drug Treatment

AT THE beginning of the twentieth century, serious cases of diabetes inevitably led to severe dehydration, coma, and death. Then it was discovered that the disease could be treated with extracts of the pancreas, the organ that releases insulin. Advances since then have progressively improved insulin treatment. Children's insulin requirements are remarkably changeable for the first year or two of their disease, so the daily dose is usually given as a regular or short-acting insulin. Small doses of regular insulin five times a day will keep the blood sugar relatively even. Quick sources of sugar must be nearby for the occasional low-blood-sugar reactions. To find a physician who uses alternative therapies and can help with the management of insulin therapy, check with the American College for Advancement in Medicine (800-532-3688) or the American Holistic Medical Association (919-787-5181).

Nutritional Support

NEITHER CONVENTIONAL nor alternative medicine currently has a cure for type 1 diabetes, but diet, exercise, and nutritional supplements can decrease insulin requirements and help prevent diabetic complications.[102] Diabetics do best eating small, frequent meals, perhaps five times a day. A wholesome diet that emphasizes legumes, vegetables, and fish, and that avoids simple and processed carbohydrates and excess fat and cholesterol, can help control blood sugar levels.

Earlier dietary recommendations involved reducing carbohydrate (from which sugar is made) and increasing fat and protein. But that diet tended to cause weight gain, and its excess fat contributed to the risk of heart disease. Fat also impairs insulin activity. A radical reversal in diabetic theory came with a landmark study reported in 1979, in which the carbohydrate intake of the diabetic was nearly doubled by substituting high-fiber complex carbohydrates for animal foods. The result was that diabetics on low doses of insulin managed to give up the drug altogether, and those on high doses substantially reduced their prescriptions.[103]

Complex carbohydrates (whole grains and beans) are digested more slowly than simple carbohydrates and are known now to actually help regulate blood sugar levels. Fiber also helps regulate glucose metabolism by delaying glucose absorption from the intestines. A high-fiber diet takes longer to be digested, and sugar from the food is absorbed over a longer period. Fiber also helps keep weight down by giving more opportunity to chew and filling the body up with fewer calories.[104] Beans and other legumes that are digested and absorbed slowly are particularly good foods for diabetics. Studies show that diets based on legumes improve diabetic glucose and insulin profiles, and that slow-release carbohydrates can help relieve the symptoms of the disease. Legumes remain the traditional staples in parts of the world like Africa and India where diabetes is uncommon.

Supplements of vitamins B_{12}, C, and E, flavonoids, magnesium, gamma linoleic acids, bilberry, and grapeseed extract can help with both managing blood sugar and preventing diabetic complications.[105]

Gymnema sylvestre, an herb used for centuries in India to support the pancreas and help regulate blood sugar, is growing in popularity with diabetics. Take it with water fifteen minutes before each meal: one capsule with a small or low-sugar meal, two with a larger or high-sugar meal.

The herb milk thistle, containing the antioxidant silymarin, has been shown to significantly drop and stabilize glucose levels without hypoglycemic episodes. The herb also helps with the utilization of insulin, reducing the amount needed.[106]

Exercise can aid in the control of diabetes by burning up excess calories and improving glucose utilization and cardiovascular performance.

Sunlight is another natural insulin. When diabetics have been exposed to sunlight treatments, their blood sugar has dropped and the sugar in their urine has decreased or disappeared. Acetone bodies also decreased or vanished. Natural sunlight seems to produce the best results.

Caution: Major changes in activity levels may require a change in drug dosage. Otherwise, increased exercise can trigger hypoglycemic episodes. Sunbathing should also be introduced gradually, since the insulinlike effect of sunlight is so dramatic that it can precipitate a hypoglycemic episode when compounded with insulin injections.[107]

DIAPER RASH, AMMONIACAL DIAPER

A RED rash in the diaper area that is confined to the skin just around the anus is probably due to a food sensitivity. Likely suspects are tomatoes, citrus fruits, and peaches. If the rash is worse in the morning, covers the diaper area, and has a strong ammonia smell, it may be due to alkaline urine.

Ammoniacal diaper is a wet diaper with the unmistakable smell of ammonia, usually greeting the parent after the child has slept all night. It can cause a contact rash, since ammonia is an irritant.

For thrush diaper rashes, see "Candidiasis."

 Natural Alternatives

FOR AMMONIACAL diaper, acidify diapers with vinegar. Try using three diapers at night and pouring an ounce of vinegar in the second diaper; this is usually enough to acidify the urine. Cloth diapers are cheaper and more environmentally sound than disposable diapers (which are choking landfills). Hanging washed diapers in the sun is sufficient to kill the germs that produce the ammonia smell.

For diaper rash, safe remedies include washing the area with certain herbal teas, including chamomile, chickweed, comfrey, elder flowers, lavender, marigold, marshmallow root, and rosemary. The herbs can also be mixed with almond oil and then strained to make a soothing rub for sore bottoms. Tinctures of Calendula, goldenseal, and myrrh are available at health food stores.[108] Homeopathic Calendula lotion may also be applied topically.

Witch hazel is an old-fashioned remedy for washing the bottom. Apple cider vinegar and lemon juice are other options for creating a more acid environment in which yeast are less able to grow. (See "Candidiasis.")

Be sure to change diapers frequently, and immediately when wet or soiled. Clean the baby's bottom with plain water and allow to dry in the air before rediapering. Allow air exposure as often as possible. Avoid plastic pants, which reduce air circulation to the area, and fabric softeners or scented detergent on diapers. Rinse cloth diapers twice to make sure all the soap is out.

DIARRHEA

DIARRHEA IS characterized by frequent, loose, watery stools, sometimes with cramping and vomiting. The occasional loose stool is normal in children, whose delicate digestive systems are more sensitive than adults' to changes in food, emotional upsets, colds, and flus. Diarrhea can be expected in children for a few days every couple of months. Frequent attacks of watery stools, however, should be investigated.

In infants and small children, diarrhea can cause dangerous dehydration; but suppressing the eliminatory process is not recommended, since the drugs can mask the signs of very serious illness and cause the retention of toxins in the body. Diarrhea represents the body's attempt to get rid of things it is better off without. Traveler's diarrhea is always caused by something ingested that the body rejects. If elimination is suppressed, the causative toxin (food, virus, or bacteria) will remain inside and prolong the upset. It can also be responsible for serious infectious diseases like typhoid and cholera. The occasional bout of diarrhea is also likely to be from food poisoning and should not be suppressed. (See "Food Poisoning.")

Call the doctor if your child has diarrhea and is under six months old; if the child seems to be dehydrated, has abdominal pain for more than two hours, has watery stools every one to two hours or more, has a fever for more than forty-eight hours, has been vomiting for more than twelve hours, refuses to eat or drink, has a rash or jaundice (yellow discoloration of the skin and whites of the eyes); if the stool has blood in it; or if the diarrhea seems to be getting worse rather than better.[109] If there is blood in the stool, a stool culture is recommended to determine if the source is bacterial. Blood in the stool could also be from hemorrhoids, sexual abuse, or a rectal tear. Dark blood the color of coffee grounds may indicate a bleeding ulcer. Although unusual in children, ulcers may be precipitated by analgesics like Advil or Motrin taken on an empty stomach. Blood in the stool can also indicate ulcerative colitis.

Children who develop diarrhea while breast-feeding may be reacting to something the mother ate: Offenders can include caffeine, herbal teas, antibiotics, and some laxatives.

Diarrhea may also be a symptom of intestinal flu, for which childcare facilities are common sources (see "Flu"). Parasites may be an another, unsuspected cause of diarrhea (see "Parasites").

 Drug Treatment

PRESCRIPTION ANTIDIARRHEA drugs are effective—in fact, they can bring bowel function to a grinding halt by drugging the nerves that trigger it—but the result may be to leave bacteria and other toxins in the body to wreak their own havoc. The drugs also contain potentially addictive narcotics. According to the FDA, most over-the-counter antidiarrheal drugs, while safer than prescription drugs, lack evidence of effectiveness.[110] Diarrhea usually goes away without drugs. **Don't give your child antidiarrhea drugs unless your pediatrician recommends them.**

The pediatrician may prescribe antibiotics if Shigella or Salmonella bacteria are found in your child's stool culture. (See "Food Poisoning.") For cautions, see "Immunity."

 ## Natural Alternatives for Children with Diarrhea

FOR SMALL children with serious diarrhea, the American Academy of Pediatrics recommends oral electrolyte solutions (Ricelyte, Pedialyte, or Rehydralyte). It does not recommend popular choices like fruit juice, water, Gatorade, and Jell-O, because their water, salt, and sugar contents are not in the proper proportions.[111] Oriental doctors recommend giving rice water (the water in which rice is boiled) to firm up the stools. It tends to constipate but contains no roughage and is therefore quite safe.

For children old enough to eat solid foods, bananas, rice, applesauce, toast, and tea are easy to digest and may help stop fluid loss. Homemade applesauce is preferred to the store-bought variety. Better yet, grate a raw, peeled, and cored apple to the consistency of applesauce. Apples contain pectin, an ingredient that helps stop diarrhea. Pectin is contained in over-the-counter antidiarrheal medicines like Kaopectate and Parapectalin, but it is destroyed by cooking.[112]

 ## Restoring and Maintaining Friendly Intestinal Flora

IN JAPAN, diarrhea in children is successfully treated with fermented dairy products to which large amounts of bifido bacteria have been added. Research has shown that beneficial bifido bacteria help control diarrhea and other intestinal problems by establishing a healthy microfloral balance. Some U.S. dairies have begun adding bifidus along with acidophilus to yogurts. In one study, children with chronic diarrhea were given traditional drug therapy, antibiotics, and special diets, yet their diarrhea persisted for as long as ten weeks. When the children were given bifido bacteria preparations, their conditions improved in three to seven days. In another study, adults with diarrhea were given bifidus-supplemented yogurt three times daily along with antibiotic treatment. After three days, the patients had less abdominal discomfort and fewer bowel movements than without bifidus supplementation.[113]

Balancing the intestines with acidophilus or bifido bacteria can help in cases of constipation, too. PB-8 by Nutrition Now is a good product for kids. It contains eight different types of acidophilus in powdered form. The same company also makes flavored chewable acidophilus tablets.

 Homeopathy and Gemmotherapy

WHILE ORAL rehydration (replenishing fluids) can prevent death from dehydration in children, it does not decrease duration or frequency of diarrhea. By contrast, a study published in 1994 in *Pediatrics* (the journal of the American Academy of Pediatrics) found that homeopathic remedies did produce a statistically significant decrease in the duration of children's diarrhea. The researchers observed that acute diarrhea is the leading cause of pediatric deaths and complications worldwide, and that inappropriate use of antibiotics for this illness is widespread in developing countries; fortunately, homeopathy, a nontoxic and accessible alternative, is also in widespread use.[114]

The first-choice homeopathic remedy for children's stomach cramps and diarrhea, particularly from intestinal flu, is Arsenicum alba. Give it in a low potency (6x, 6c, 30x, or 30c) at a dosage of two pills two to three times daily at the onset of symptoms. It acts by inducing symptoms, so there could be a slight homeopathic aggravation. (See Introduction.)

For food poisoning, a single dose of homeopathic Salmonella 200x will often relieve even severe cramping and nausea. Arsenicum alba 6x is another useful homeopathic remedy for cramps, nausea, vomiting, and pain resulting from food poisoning. The dosage is two pills every fifteen minutes, up to six doses. Traveler's diarrhea can be relieved with Arsenicum alba or with the homeopathic remedy Worms by CompliMed or Ver by Deseret.

Gemmotherapy is another safe and effective alternative for diarrhea or spasmodic colitis: Wineberry is a gentle way to slow elimination and soothe the bowel.

For other remedies, see "Stomachache," "Intestinal Flu."

 What to Avoid

IF DIARRHEA strikes your child after eating a food that leaves others at the table unaffected, the problem may be a food allergy or intolerance. To pinpoint the problem, feed your child a bland diet, then add suspicious foods back in one by one until likely offenders are located. (See "Allergies.") To replace lost fluids, offer plenty of water or juice diluted with water (but not heavily sugared drinks).

Milk products can aggravate an active case of diarrhea even in children who are not normally allergic to them and should be avoided; dairy products contain lactose, which is hard to digest. Also avoid caffeinated beverages. Drugs can cause or aggravate diarrhea as well: Antibiotics are lead offenders.

DIPHTHERIA

DIPHTHERIA IS a serious and highly contagious bacterial infection characterized by a gray cast to the throat, hoarseness, malaise, fever (not usually above 102 degrees), and formation of a white, patchy, grayish fur or membrane on the tonsils. The disease begins in the throat and respiratory tract. A thick membrane forms on the tonsils, in the nose, and on the windpipe; and the throat is sore and swollen. Breathing becomes difficult due to obstructed airways. Weakness, heart failure, and death may follow. The disease is much less common than it once was, but whether this is because of the mandatory use of the DPT (diphtheria/pertussis/tetanus) vaccine or because of better sanitation is debated. Diphtheria has been known to occur in immunized persons, and the disease was already on the wane before vaccinating for it became widespread. (See "Immunizations.")

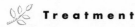 **Treatment**

THE ANTIBIOTIC erythromycin is the conventional treatment for diphtheria. A tracheotomy (making a hole in the trachea) may be performed if breathing is seriously obstructed.

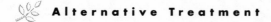 **Alternative Treatment**

DIPHTHERIA IS a serious condition requiring professional medical care, but homeopathic remedies can help relieve symptoms. For cases in which a membrane forms in the throat, the remedy is Kali bichrom. For cases involving a shiny, red, and painful throat, the remedy is Belladonna 200, taken every two hours. For a sudden attack of diphtheria, the remedy is Mercurius cyanatus.

DOG BITES (See Animal Bites)

DOWN'S SYNDROME

THIS IS a genetic condition resulting in mental retardation. Other common features include short stature, soft muscles, and extra eyelid folds. Children with Down's syndrome tend to be very affectionate and cheerful and can be a joy to a loving, nurturing family despite their limitations. Extra vitamins, minerals, and sometimes thyroid hormone can help speed their slowed development.

Acupuncture can also help. Dr. Dung Tran, an Oriental-medicine practitioner in Canada, has had quite remarkable success with Down's syndrome. If children are less than one year old when treatment is begun, Dr. Tran states that his treatments may make them very close to normal. Author Dr. Walker saw an eight-month-old baby who was much better after this treatment, and was dramatically improved a year later. Dr. Tran may be reached at 613-729-1154.

DRY SKIN (See Dermatitis)

DYSLEXIA

DYSLEXIA IS a condition in which children have trouble reading with comprehension. The condition occurs in about 5 percent of the population, is more common in boys, and seems to have a genetic component. It is often associated with hyperactivity, either because the child cannot settle down and concentrate or because frustration with his reading difficulty makes him hyperactive.

Dyslexia is more common in schools employing the Look-and-Say method, which teaches by whole words ("See Spot. See Spot run."). Phonics, teaching the child to identify and sound out parts of words, is the preferred method when dyslexia is suspected. There is evidence that children who were placed in walkers as infants and were not allowed to crawl and creep may have more trouble learning to read. (See "Crawling.") Sugar and junk food have been associated with hyperactivity and should be kept to a minimum in the diet of a child who has trouble concentrating. (See "ADD.")

 ## Alternative Approaches

DYSLEXIA IS conventionally attributed to a central lesion in the brain and is considered a handicap, but in *The Gift of Dyslexia: Why Some of the Smartest People Can't Read . . . and How They Can Learn,* Ronald Davis and Eldon Braun argue that the condition is a gift. They note that a number of geniuses were dyslexic, including Albert Einstein, Thomas Edison, Alexander Graham Bell, Leonardo da Vinci, Walt Disney, Winston Churchill, and Woodrow Wilson. The authors maintain that these people were geniuses not in spite of but because of their dyslexia, which took the focus off the details of words and presented the larger picture. The authors list these gifted traits of dyslexics: They think mainly in pictures instead of words; are highly intuitive and insightful; can use the brain's ability to alter and create perceptions; are highly aware of the environment; are more curious than average; think and perceive multidimensionally (using all the senses); can experience thought as reality; and have vivid imaginations. "These eight basic abilities, if not suppressed, invalidated, or destroyed by parents or the educational process," write Davis and Braun, "will result in two characteristics: higher than normal intelligence, and extraordinary creative abilities." The authors present techniques for teaching dyslexics to read and overcome clumsiness.[115]

EAR INFECTIONS (OTITIS MEDIA)

MIDDLE-EAR INFECTION (otitis media) has reached epidemic proportions among American children, despite aggressive drug treatment. Parents spend more than $1 billion annually on the condition, which has been called the bread and butter of the pediatrician.[116] Chronic middle-ear effusion (fluid in the ears) underlies the most frequently performed operations of childhood—myringotomy (surgical incision of the eardrum, with or without the insertion of tubes), tonsillectomy, and adenoidectomy. Parents sometimes elect myringotomy because they're afraid that chronic fluid in the ears will reduce hearing and impair learning. But recent studies show that the effectiveness of these operations is very limited, and that they should be reserved only for children who are severely affected. They can mean further trauma to the eardrum, prolonging the time required for the ear to heal, and they do not shorten the duration of pain. In most cases, the condition eventually clears by itself without surgery, presumably because the skull and eustachian tubes have grown.[117]

 Drug Treatment

ANTIBIOTICS ARE standard treatment for ear infections, but the ailment often fails to respond even to repeated courses of the drugs.[118] The majority of ear infections are caused by viruses, for which antibiotics don't work; and the widespread use of antibiotics has led to the widespread development of antibiotic-resistant strains of bacteria.[119] A landmark Swedish study involving 2,145 patients showed that ear infections did not go away any faster when treated with antibiotics, and children treated with them were 30 percent more likely to have a recurrence of the infection. The drugs depress the immunological response to bacteria, preventing the development of natural antibodies and interfering with the development of natural immunity. They also permit overgrowth by resistant Candida microbes, which then produce toxins that can weaken the immune system and further reduce the child's resistance.[120] (See "Candidiasis.") Results of this Swedish study were confirmed in a later study reported in *The New England Journal of Medicine,* finding that neither the popular antibiotic amoxicillin nor a decongestant-antihistamine provided any advantage over no drugs at all.[121] Other studies of otitis media with fluid in the ears have found that the majority of cases resolved themselves by the following month without treatment.[122]

 ## Homeopathic Alternatives

THE BEST course of action is to let your child's ear infections resolve naturally. While you are waiting, try natural remedies to ease ear pain. Particularly good is Mullein Oil Ear Drops. Mullein is a strong painkiller with narcotic properties, but it does not produce the light-headedness or psychological aberrations of narcotic drugs. Applied directly in the ear, it quiets irritated nerves, relieves pain, and soothes inflammation. Other helpful herbs are echinacea and elderberry.

An excellent homeopathic combination popular in France is a product called ABC. The letters stand for Aconite, Belladonna, and Chamomile, the three main homeopathic remedies for soothing ear pain and promoting healing. Given as often as every ten or fifteen minutes at the onset of pain (or in young children when they start pulling on their ears), it can eliminate ear pain with as few as two doses. ABC is available in the U.S. from MarcoPharma International, or its ingredients can be purchased separately and taken together. Other good products are Earache Pain Relief by Natra-Bio and Chamomilla Complex by BHI. Give one pill every hour for severe pain, or one pill three times daily.

An effective home remedy for ear pain is to squeeze a few drops of fresh onion juice directly into the ear using a garlic press. Cotton can be applied afterward to hold the juice in. Fresh-squeezed garlic oil, warmed on a spoon over the stove, is another option.

Homeopathic writer Kathy Arnos recommends acidophilus and daily flaxseed oil for children with ear infections. She also looks at the teeth of a moody, irritable child, since many childhood ear problems are related to teething. Homeopathic remedies that can speed the eruption of teeth include Calc carb 200x (give three pills three times in one day, then stop) and Calc phos 6x (three pills two times daily for one week).

A product by Child Life called Essential Fatty Acids has been found to help in cases of ear infection. It comes in a liquid form that is easy for kids to take.

Ear candling, in which a waxed paper cylinder is placed in the ear and burned at the protruding end to draw out wax and infection, is a solution for relieving ear pain that is controversial but growing in popularity. Mothers report that when ear candles have been used on children with ear problems, the pain disappears immediately. See "Hearing Impairment."

ECZEMA (See Dermatitis)

ELECTRIC SHOCK (See Shock, Burns)

ENVIRONMENTAL ILLNESS, LIVER STAGNATION

CHILDREN AS well as adults can suffer from the generalized liver stagnation sometimes called "environmental illness." Children with this condition are generally tired and run-down, get frequent colds, and may have allergies and skin afflictions. The problem results when the liver has become so overburdened with accumulated toxins that it can't keep up. Unsuspected immune system assailants may include pesticides sprayed in the house, on the lawn, or on a nearby golf course; formaldehyde and other chemical fumes from the upholstery in a new car, new carpeting, paint, fire retardants in a new mattress, or dry-cleaning fluid; petrochemicals in perfumes, dyes, plastics, or synthetic rubber; chlorine in swimming pools; metals and plastics in dental materials; and molds and fungi growing in damp environments. Adults who are continually ill and run-down frequently report having been exposed to environmental toxins as children. Cases known to the authors include a woman who lived next to a golf course and played on its pesticide-laden grass as a child; a woman raised on Three Mile Island; and a woman whose father was a carpenter and left the stained furniture in her bedroom because there was nowhere else in the house to put it. Continual exposure to environmental toxins causes them to accumulate in the system and overwhelm the body and the immune system. The diagnosis is established when detoxification measures reverse the problem.

 ## Detoxifying Chemical Toxins

HOMEOPATHIC REMEDIES can neutralize chemical toxins. A new line of products has been designed specifically for detoxifying particular chemicals in the body. CompliMed makes one that includes Enviro-Pest for pesticides, Enviro-Chem for chemicals, and Enviro-Met for heavy metals. Deseret makes Addiclenz for sensitivity to food additives, Enviro-I and Enviro-II for environmental chemicals, Chemtox for chemicals in general, and a line of remedies called phenolics for specific chemical sensitivities (such as Acetaldehyde for formaldehyde sensitivity—the child who reacts to new carpet or car upholstery). Molecular Biologicals makes a remedy called Household Chemicals for people allergic to household cleaners. Apex makes ExChem for chemical sensitivity. Nature Knows makes Chloroflor for chlorine-bleach detoxification (good for use after swimming in a chlorinated swimming pool).

Chlorine Sensitivity Reversed

A mother complained of bad acne in her nine-year-old daughter, who seemed too young for the problem. The girl's acne was aggravated whenever she went swimming. A homeopathic specifically formulated for eliminating chlorine from the system worked to clear up the girl's complexion, except on the days that she swam. The mother then started giving her the remedy before and after swimming and reported that the girl had no further acne problems.

 ## Detoxifying Molds and Fungi

AN INCREASING but unrecognized problem is sensitivity to molds and fungi, which can linger after the rainy season and blow into the house from musty basements through heating and air-conditioning systems. The black mold that grows on walls is highly toxic to children and was linked in a recent study to brain damage in infants. (See "Asthma.") There is no known conventional treatment. Homeopathic remedies designed to address the problem include Fungisode, Fungotox I, and Fungotox II, all by Molecular Biologicals, and Mold/Yeast/Dust by CompliMed.

Baffling Family Ailment Reversed

A mother complained that her whole family seemed to be continually sick. Despite the usual preventive measures, Sam, her nine-month-old baby, got repeated colds. On questioning, the mother said they were living in a condominium converted from an old hotel in Sun Valley. In its dilapidated former state, the roof had leaked water into the walls. The walls had been painted, but black mold was still evident. Worse, the family was using a humidifier every day, which wet the windows, making the baby's room a breeding ground for toxic molds and fungi. Mold and Fungus by Molecular Biologicals was recommended to the family, and all felt better after taking it. They finally broke their lease and moved, and reported having never felt healthier.

 ### Detoxifying the Liver

THE LIVER must break down all the toxins that come into the body before they are excreted; it has its work cut out for it just detoxifying the normal products of metabolism. When extraordinary environmental toxins and drugs are added to that load, it can get so overwhelmed that it cannot do its job. Chinese doctors say the internal movements of the body then stagnate. The Chinese patent remedy for moving liver stagnation is Hsiao Yao Wan.

Particular foods can also help detoxify the system by stimulating drainage of the liver. Foods high in inositol and choline help the liver eliminate excess fat, while foods high in sulfur and selenium act as antioxidants. Good choices include watercress, mustard greens, red and black radishes, wheat-grass juice, dandelions, parsley, apples, artichokes, beets and beet greens, carrots, brussels sprouts, horseradish, garlic, cabbage, cranberries, Swiss chard, kale, and celery.

The Liver Cleanse Diet

THE FOLLOWING liver detox program has been modified for children. It can be continued for four or five days:

1. Each morning, the child's routine should begin with one teaspoonful of lemon juice squeezed into warm water, sweetened with honey if desired.

2. Encourage the child to drink the juice of fresh mixed greens (parsley, celery, carrot) at least twice a day. If you can't find these drinks or make them yourself, give chlorophyll in water or juice, two to four ounces daily, mixed in apple juice to sweeten. Also have the child drink unfiltered apple juice throughout the day.

3. The diet should consist of only whole, fresh foods—no preservatives, coloring, or fillers (all found in processed foods). Emphasize green vegetables, which stimulate the liver to release and process toxins. Limit protein to thirty grams a day.

4. Have the child drink at least thirty-two ounces (four glasses) of distilled water daily while on the detox diet. (Distilled water isn't recommended for more than seven days, since it contains no electrolytes and depletes them in the body.)

5. Encourage sedentary children to get more exercise.

EPIGLOTTITIS (See Croup)

EPILEPSY (See Seizures)

EYE INFECTION, EYE IRRITATION, PINKEYE, CONJUNCTIVITIS, STYES

CONJUNCTIVITIS, OR pinkeye, is an inflammation of the thin, clear layer of tissue covering the outside surface of the white of the eyeball. It can be caused by bacteria, a virus, an allergy, a blocked tear duct, a foreign body in the eye, or a chemical irritant. The latter may include the silver nitrate routinely dropped in the eyes of newborns to prevent contracting gonococcal conjunctivitis when the baby passes through the birth canal from a mother who has this infection in her genitalia.

Infectious conjunctivitis is caused by a virus or bacteria. Contaminated swimming pools are a common source of infection. Bacterial conjunctivitis causes only mild discomfort but can produce copious discharge and redness. It typically begins in one eye but can move to the other. It shows as a green or yellow purulent discharge that usually glues the eyelids together. Viral conjunctivitis may involve a clear watery discharge and is often associated with colds. It usually includes fever, malaise, redness, and copious discharge from the eye.

Other common minor eye ailments include styes (bacterial infection of the tiny glands at the base of the eyelid), dry eyes, torn corneas, and redness or tiredness from overwork.

 Conventional Treatment

PINKEYE USUALLY goes away by itself in a few days. If it doesn't, antibiotic ointments are commonly prescribed, but they will have no effect on the more common viral conjunctivitis, since antibiotics work only on bacteria; and antibiotics are hazardous for other reasons. (See "Immunity.") Besides antibiotic eyedrops or ointments, steroid or sulfacetamide eyedrops or ointments may be prescribed. All can have side effects. Corticosteroids and corticosteroid/antibiotic combinations are also hazardous. Corticosteroids suppress inflammation; and when inflammation is reduced, resistance is lowered and secondary infections can occur. The drugs can also cause glaucoma and cataracts.[123]

Over-the-counter eye medications that remove redness can have unwanted side effects as well. Cases of blindness have actually been reported from excess use.[124] Drugs dropped into the eyes reach the general circulation; and since the contact time with the eye is often only a fraction of a minute, eye medications are highly concentrated. They drain rapidly back into the mucous membranes of the nose, where they can enter the bloodstream and reach the heart, lungs, and other organs without being detoxified.[125]

 Natural Alternatives

FOR PINKEYE, safe, effective homeopathic remedies can clear the condition in just a couple of days. Eye by BHI is particularly good. It contains several homeopathic medicines, including Euphrasia, which clears redness. Also good is Optique by Boiron, containing homeopathic Euphrasia and Calendula. These individually packaged eyedrops remain sterile and contain no preservatives.

All antioxidants are beneficial for the eyes. They include alpha-lipoic acid, coenzyme Q10, cysteine, glutathione, melatonin, selenium, superoxide dismutase, vitamin A and beta-carotene, vitamins C and E, zinc, and oligomeric proanthocyanids (OPCs). OPCs are powerful antioxidants found in grape seeds and pine bark (pycnogenol). Most of these antioxidants are contained in a combination nutritional product good for vision problems called Ocudyne II. The capsule is quite large for children but can be opened and the contents mixed in juice.

Herbs high in antioxidants include bilberry, ginkgo biloba, and green tea. Bilberry has been shown to increase night vision. The herb eyebright (Euphrasia) is also good for any eye problem—pinkeye, tired eyes, and puffy eyes. It comes in several forms, including capsules, bulk herbs, and tinctures. It can be drunk as a tea, and the tea bags can be placed on the eyes.

Full-spectrum lighting is important for the eyes. Glass windows and lenses filter out beneficial components of the sun's rays. Dr. Jacob Lieberman recommends spending at least an hour each day outdoors, regardless of the weather. It need not be in the sun—being in the shade or on a screened porch is fine—but for this therapy to work, sunglasses, prescription glasses, contact lenses, and suntan lotion should not be used. Direct solar rays between ten A.M. and two P.M. are best avoided. For sunscreen issues and alternatives, see "Sunburn."

FEAR OF THE DARK (See Night Terrors)

FEVER

FEVER IS one of the most common symptoms prompting parents to bring their young children to the doctor. A common fear is that fever will cause brain damage, but a careful review of the literature by several investigators has failed to confirm this adverse effect. The only possible exceptions were in cases of meningitis or encephalitis, but the relationship was uncertain, since those conditions can cause brain damage independently of fever. In any case, fever won't cause brain damage below 108 degrees, and temperatures that high are extremely rare.[126] Another concern is that fevers can provoke seizures in children who are prone to them. However, drugs aren't usually effective in preventing this type of seizure, since by the time the fever is recognized, the seizure is already in full swing. Fortunately, these seizures (which are not related to epilepsy) are harmless.[127]

The Greek physician Hippocrates, traditionally regarded as the father of medicine, considered fever a therapeutic process designed to "cook out" invaders. His attitude prevailed until the twentieth century, when aspirin was introduced. By the turn of that century, drug companies were promoting aspirin for its ability to reduce fever as well as pain, which seemed to go together. Ultimately, mass advertising turned public sentiment against this natural cleansing process, but new research supports Hippocrates. A little fever, it seems, does a body good. Studies show that fever cripples many temperature-sensitive viruses. In laboratory experiments, artificially induced fevers have decreased the death rate among infected animals, while lowering their temperatures has *increased* the death rate. In European hydrotherapies, fever is intentionally induced for its cleansing effects. Fever evidently fights disease by means of a substance called interleukin1 (IL1), which is released from white blood cells when a foreign agent invades the blood. Fever raises the thermostat in the hypothalamus, probably by activating prostaglandins. Aspirin works by suppressing prostaglandins. IL1 speeds the production of the immune system's T cells, which augment natural killer-cell activity. When the temperature rises from 98.6 to 102 degrees Fahrenheit, T-cell production increases by as much as twenty times. When aspirin is given to rabbits in doses sufficient to prevent fever, the killing activity of their neutrophils (a type of white blood cell) is inhibited. High body temperatures also strengthen the effect of interferon, a natural protein that combats viruses.[128]

Get a doctor's advice for any fever over 103 degrees or for one above 100 degrees that lasts more than three days, especially if accompanied by a very sore throat. In a pregnant woman, a high fever can be harmful to the fetus during the first three months of pregnancy.

 ## The Conventional Approach

ASPIRIN WAS long the standard treatment for reducing fevers, until aspirin treatment of viral infections was linked to Reye's syndrome, an often fatal disease. The brain damage commonly attributed to the natural fever process seems in these cases to have been caused by the drugs given to treat it. (See "Reye's Syndrome.")

Because of this serious aspirin risk, acetaminophen (Tylenol and others) is now generally recommended for reducing fever in children. Aspirin, acetaminophen, and ibuprofen are all about equally effective in reducing fever, but acetaminophen is considered the safest. There is still a question, however, whether fever should be reduced at all. In one study, sixty-eight children with chicken pox were given either acetaminophen or a placebo four times a day for four days. On the second day of treatment, children in the acetominophen-treated group were more active than those in the placebo group. But on the fourth day, the treated children itched more, and their chicken pox took a day longer to scab over. The data suggested that the effects of fever were actually beneficial in fighting off the virus, and that fever should be allowed to run its course.[129]

Some pediatricians routinely treat fevers with antibiotics, even before they have laboratory evidence of bacterial infection. But most fevers will go away by themselves without treatment; and even if they don't, antibiotics won't usually help, since only 3 to 15 percent of fevers are caused by bacteria, and antibiotics are not effective on viral infections. A study in *The New England Journal of Medicine* concluded that routine treatment of high fever in small children with standard oral doses of antibiotics (in that case, amoxicillin) was unwarranted, except when actual laboratory evidence of a bacterial infection justified it.[130]

 Natural Remedies

ALTHOUGH FEVERS serve beneficial functions, they can be uncomfortable and can lead to febrile seizures. To reduce fever and its symptoms, homeopathic remedies are the ideal first choice of treatment, since they do not interfere with the natural efforts of the body. Homeopaths treat the whole symptom picture, not just the fever. Here are some common symptom complexes and their appropriate homeopathic remedies:

Belladonna 6x to 30c: For the child who is restless, with a very hot face, who feels better with cold applications. Give the remedy every fifteen minutes for two hours, or until the fever has come down.

Belladonna 200x or 1M: For febrile seizures (seizures triggered by fever). Give two to three pills every two hours.

Ferrum phos 6x to 30c: For the child with a temperature but no localized symptoms. Give two to three pills at intervals of fifteen to sixty minutes as needed, up to five doses.

Aconitum 6x to 30c: For the fever that comes on suddenly, often after exposure to wind or cold. The child is usually thirsty. Give two pills every fifteen minutes as needed, up to five doses.

Fever Reducer by Boericke & Tafel is an effective homeopathic combination product.

Herbal remedies are also available. Herbs for Kids makes one called Temp Assure for treating fever, headache, and other symptoms of the first onset of the flu. It contains the herbs peppermint, elderberry, and yarrow. Chinese herbal formulas for treating fever include:

Zhong Gan Ling by Zand: For a cold with fever. K'an Herbs also makes one by the same name.

Liu Shen Wan: For fever with strep throat. This formula has been known to eliminate severe strep throat symptoms in only a few hours.

Antiphlogistic Tablets: An effective Chinese patent remedy for sore throat or tonsillitis accompanied by fever.

For the case of a child having febrile seizures, see "Seizures."

FEVER BLISTERS (See Cold Sores)

FLU, INFLUENZA

THE FLU is a very contagious upper respiratory infection caused by the influenza virus. Symptoms include generalized achiness with a runny nose, sneezing, cough, headache, sore throat, weakness, chills, fever, and possibly vomiting and diarrhea. Flu epidemics hit most frequently in the winter or early spring. Child-care facilities are common sources, as children are not usually excluded unless they are feverish or lethargic. Facilities should be checked by parents for proper diapering and hand-washing practices. See also "Intestinal Flu," "Stomachache," "Diarrhea."

 Conventional Treatment

BECAUSE THE flu is caused by a virus, antibiotics will not cure it. The usual treatment is rest with plenty of fluids and a painkiller like Tylenol. **Caution: Children with flu should not take aspirin due to the risk of Reye's syndrome.** See "Fever," "Reye's Syndrome."

For prevention, flu shots are heavily promoted; but Julian Whitaker, M.D., warns strongly against this prophylactic measure. The flu shot is specific for certain strains, and will not work on epidemics of unanticipated strains. Moreover, tampering with the immune system is risky business. Unlike vaccinations for childhood diseases, in which a single course is considered good for a lifetime, flu shots must be repeated every year. According to some studies, 50 percent of people who get the shots have complications, and for a small percentage, they can be life-threatening. Many people report getting a bad case of the flu right after the shot, suggesting a causal link. In anticipation of a swine-flu epidemic in 1976, a vaccine aimed at that scourge caused thousands of cases of Guillain-Barré syndrome, a very serious neurological disease that can be fatal; yet the swine-flu epidemic never hit. There are safer and more effective ways to prevent flu.[131]

 Natural Alternatives

IN A Canadian study, taking vitamins and minerals cut the incidence of adult sick days from flu by nearly 50 percent—more than with the flu shot, without side effects or risks.[132]

Elderberry extract (Sambucus nigra) is a very popular herbal remedy for colds and flu. Rather than merely suppressing the body's eliminatory mechanisms, elderberry extract has been shown to actually halt the spread of the virus. A recent study suggests it can significantly reduce the length and severity of flu symptoms.[133] An extract of the herb was shown in an Israeli study to cut recovery times in half.[134] Elderberry comes in chewable flavors for children.

Other herbs good for preventing and treating flus and colds include echinacea, garlic, goldenseal, ginger, peppermint, and olive-leaf extract. (For cautions about echinacea, see "Colds.")

Homeopathic remedies are also effective. Homeopathic Oscillococcinum, the largest-selling flu remedy in France, was shown in a clinical study to be significantly better than a placebo in treating the flu.[135] The remedy comes in a package containing six little tubes of tiny granules. The best way to use it is to take one tube at the onset of symptoms, then mix another tube into a glass of water and sip it slowly over the next six hours. One tube may also be taken every week during flu season as a preventative instead of flu shots.

Dolisos Cold and Flu Solution Plus is a cheaper and more comprehensive homeopathic alternative that is good to use at the first sign of flu. The dosage is one tablet every fifteen minutes for the first hour, then one pill four times a day.

The German homeopathic company Staufen also makes a number of effective influenza remedies specific for each year. Comparable series therapy is available in the United States from Deseret. Other homeopathic options are Influenza and Viral CM by CompliMed, and Virus and Virus Combination by Deseret.

Sleep, fluids, and stress reduction are important. For additional remedies to boost the immune system, see "Immunity," "Colds."

FOOD ALLERGIES (See Allergies)

FOOD POISONING, SALMONELLA

SYMPTOMS OF food poisoning, including nausea, vomiting, and diarrhea, usually appear within hours of eating infected foods. Many strains of bacteria can be responsible. Most common is salmonella, a bacterial infection that can cause fever, vomiting, and diarrhea. It gives the stools a characteristic rotten-egg odor. The highly publicized deaths of children who ate meat at a popular fast-food chain in Seattle were traced to another common bacteria, *E. coli*. Sometimes the infectious agent is never known. Antibiotic overuse is blamed for the increasing incidence and seriousness of food poisoning.

 Conventional Treatment

ANTIBIOTICS ARE the conventional remedy for food poisoning, but antibiotic-resistant strains of the responsible bacteria are on the increase. Health officials are now urging doctors to avoid using antibiotics to treat children who complain of gastrointestinal ailments that could be caused by *E. coli* infection, since the drugs have been found to significantly increase the risk of contracting a life-threatening illness from the bacteria.[136] Antibiotics are routinely fed to animals to increase their growth, giving antibiotic-resistant strains an opportunity to develop. If one of these strains is ingested when a child or adult happens to be taking an antibiotic, the drug will wipe out all but the resistant bacteria. These bacteria will then take over in the gut, resulting in a "superinfection" that can be life-threatening.[137]

 Natural Alternatives

HOMEOPATHY PROVIDES effective natural alternatives. Particularly good is a German homeopathic remedy in ampule form called Salmonella by Staufen. Comparable series therapy is available from the American company Deseret.

Salmonella by Hanna Kroeger is a good combination homeopathic product.

Arsenicum alba 6c to 30c is an effective single remedy for salmonella and other food poisonings with cramping, diarrhea, and nausea. Take two pills every hour for four hours.

Also see "Stomachaches, "Diarrhea," and "Nausea."

FRACTURES (See Bones, Broken or Fractured)

FUNGAL INFECTIONS: ATHLETE'S FOOT, JOCK ITCH, RINGWORM, SWIMMER'S EAR

ATHLETE'S FOOT and *jock itch* are fungal infections that tend to get picked up or bred in gyms (hence their names). Athlete's foot manifests as a rash or patch of cracked, scaly, very itchy skin on the foot. Jock itch is the same fungus spread to the groin.

Ringworm is a fungal infection of the scalp, skin, and nails. It is not actually caused by a worm. It is very contagious and can also be contracted in gyms, or at camp or from close contact with an infected animal or human. Ringworm of the body (tinea corporis) is very common in children and is usually found on the exposed skin surfaces—face, neck, forearms, and lower legs. It is round or oval, scaly, and slightly pink, with a raised border as it grows peripherally. Tiny vesicles may dot this border. The center may be almost clear once the lesion is well developed.

Ringworm of the scalp (tinea capitis) is a fungal invasion of the hair shaft producing a brittleness that causes the hair to break, leaving a well-circumscribed patch of stubble. Rarely is there any skin inflammation or itch associated with this infection. Some types produce only a scaly patch; others invade the skin, producing a violently sensitive, swollen sore or multiple crusts. Most are spread by human contact. The infection is usually found on the back of the head, where the child has leaned against a chair on which some infected hairs were left by the preceding occupant.

Swimmer's ear is a fungal infection of the skin of the ear canal caused by the retention of moisture in the outer ear canal. The moist condition encourages infection. One clue to fungal infection is an odor like dirty socks. The child's ears will also itch.

Fungal infection can affect other parts of the body, particularly the toenails and fingernails. In children, fungal infections are usually confined to the skin, hair, or nails; but some fungi will invade the inner body (actinomycosis, blastomycosis, cryptococcosis, sporotrichosis, histoplasmosis, coccidioidomycosis). Difficult-to-treat fungus cases are generally a sign of systemic infection with *Candida albicans,* indicating that the immune system is impaired. (See "Candidiasis.")

Conventional Treatment

ANTIFUNGAL CREAMS like Tinactin or Lotrimin are the conventional remedies for athlete's foot and jock itch. For the feet, the recommended procedure is to soak for ten minutes in warm salt water before applying the cream. These creams are effective but may cause local irritation, and the effects are often only temporary. Over-the-counter antihistamines are also given for symptomatic relief.

Topical drugs are ineffective against nail fungus, so oral systemic drugs must be prescribed. Until recently, the drugs used were griseofulvin and ketoconazole; but side effects ranging from annoying to serious, along with a high relapse rate, made doctors reluctant to prescribe them. A new line of broad-spectrum oral antifungal agents, promoted as working quickly and safely on fungal conditions, has now hit the market, including itraconazole (Sporanox), terbinafine (Lamasil), and fluconazole (Diflucan).[138] But new research indicates that these drugs, too, can be hazardous; and they're very expensive and require months of use. The popular Diflucan has been linked to a remote but serious risk of liver damage. (See "Candidiasis.")

Conventional treatment for ringworm of the scalp is with a four- to six-week course of griseofulvin taken orally. Topical antifungal medicines are ineffective. Diflucan, Sporanox, and Lamasil are effective but not yet approved by the FDA.

For swimmer's ear, first wash out the debris in the ear canal; then insert an ointment, cream, or drops containing antibacterial and antifungal drugs.

Natural Alternatives

TEA TREE oil is an anti-infective that is more natural and less toxic than drugs. For athlete's foot, apply several drops to the feet twice a day. Part of the problem is that the fungus gets inside the shoes, recontaminating the feet, so treat the shoes with tea tree oil spray or powder as well. Tea tree oil also comes as eardrops for fungal infections of the ear and as a mouthwash and toothpaste for treating fungal infections of the mouth. For fungal infections of the scalp, it can be added to shampoo. (See "Head Lice.")

Another nondrug anti-infective is colloidal silver (silver suspended in a liquid medium). It can be used topically as a spray or taken orally if the spray is insufficient to eliminate symptoms. It works in difficult cases, but like antifungal drugs, it doesn't necessarily cure the problem for good; and while it doesn't have serious reported side effects like the drugs, silver is a heavy metal with unknown long-term effects.

Other natural agents that effectively eliminate fungi and parasites without side effects are oral grapefruit-seed extract (by NutriBiotic) and a combination Chinese product called Wu oil (applied topically). For swimmer's ear, use grapefruit-seed eardrops or MSM eardrops. For nail fungus, use Wu oil for cleaning under the nails with a scrub brush.

Homeopathic fungus remedies can boost the immune system enough to allow it to eliminate fungal infections permanently. Effective options include FNG by Deseret; and Fungisode and Molds, Yeast, and Dust by Molecular Biologicals.

Prevention

RECOMMENDED MEASURES for preventing athlete's foot and jock itch include drying the groin and feet thoroughly with a towel or with a blow dryer set on low (if using a towel, dry the feet last to avoid spreading the fungus), putting antifungal powder in shoes and on the feet, showering in sandals, changing shoes and socks frequently, and (for boys) wearing loose-fitting cotton boxers rather than tight-fitting briefs.[139]

For swimmer's ear, use rubbing alcohol on a thin swab of cotton as a drying agent, after the debris has been washed out and after each swim session or hair wash. Use a hair dryer set on low to blow the ears dry after swimming or showering.

For prevention and treatment of Candida, see "Candidiasis." For reversing sensitivity to molds and fungi in the environment, see "Environmental Illness."

GAS (See Stomachache)

GLUTEN INTOLERANCE (See Celiac Disease)

GROWING PAINS (See Muscle Cramps)

HAY FEVER (See Allergies)

HEADACHES

HEADACHES IN children are more likely to indicate an organic disease than tension, worry, or neurosis. Most commonly they are associated with fevers of viral origin. Children under eight are usually unable to describe the pain's severity or type (throbbing, steady, dull, sharp). The parents can only infer a headache by the child's undue lethargy, furrowed brow, scalp rubbing, or ear pulling.

Tension headaches are dull and persistent, affecting both sides of the head. They can be a symptom of anxiety, stress, physical tension, lack of sleep, overconsumption of caffeine, fever, hypoglycemia, drug side effects, dehydration, or trauma. Eye strain can also cause tension headaches. A child who needs glasses is liable to avoid reading to avoid the headache.

Migraine headaches most often appear only one side of the head. They are severe, recurrent headaches typically accompanied by nausea, vomiting, "auras" (visual disturbances), light-headedness, intolerance to light, and numbness or tingling in the head or arms. In adults, attacks last four to seventy-two hours and occur an average of one to four times a month. Heredity is a factor. One or both parents of most migraine sufferers also had them.

In children, migraine headaches are uncommon and are usually associated with vomiting, to the point that the head pain is almost forgotten; or the pain may be all over the head and not just on one side as is typical in an adult. This condition, called *cyclic vomiting,* also seems to be genetic. The vomiting may be triggered by some stressor and continues for twenty-four hours, leaving the child pale and weak. Evidently these children begin to burn fat for energy, resulting in acetonemia (an acid condition). The body compensates by vomiting, which gets rid of stomach acid but does not seem to stop the condition from running its course. These children may grow up to have the more typical migraine headaches.

A similar headache associated with abnormal brain waves is the *epileptic equivalent.* It comes on suddenly and is associated with pallor. A giveaway clue is that the child falls asleep afterward as if the nervous system were exhausted.

Food sensitivities are a frequent cause of headaches in children. Common allergenic foods include chocolate, corn, pork, milk, nuts, fish, and eggs. Monosodium glutamate (MSG), food preservatives, amino acids such as tyramine, and nitrates can all affect the blood vessels and precipitate headaches. A good plan is for the parent to make a diet calendar, listing all the foods consumed by the child in the three to twelve hours preceding a headache. Repeated patterns help pinpoint culprits.

Headaches can also be caused by a misaligned bite. Temporo-mandibular joint dysfunction (TMJ) is a dental condition that results from irritation of the disk connecting the jaw to the skull. If this is the problem, before succumbing to expensive mouth reconstruction, have the child try making a studied effort to relax the jaw. Tension can throw off the bite, resulting in headaches. A dentist can also fit the child with a mouthpiece to wear at night to relieve jaw tension.[140]

Sinus trouble can also cause headaches. When it is severe enough to have that effect, it will usually afford other clues, including purulent discharge, fever, and tenderness to bone pressure at the sinus site.

Sudden severe headaches can signal something more serious, such as hemorrhage or bleeding inside the brain. A severe headache with stiff neck and fever may indicate meningitis or meningoencephalitis. A brain tumor or blood clot stretching the meninges would also cause headache pain. Seek medical advice.

 ## Conventional Treatment

IN ADULTS, most tension headaches are treated with over-the-counter analgesics (aspirin, acetaminophen, ibuprofen); but these drugs can have side effects, and children should not be given aspirin due to the risk of Reye's syndrome. Try natural alternatives before analgesics.

For migraine, children are usually given phenobartibal. Imitrex, a new drug that is popular for treating adult migraines, is also sometimes given to young people.[141] By 1995 Imitrex was being used by more than two million sufferers worldwide, but the FDA had received 3,526 voluntary reports by then of suspected side effects, including 83 deaths and at least 273 life-threatening complications.[142] Nausea and dizziness are other side effects.

 ## Natural Alternatives

FOR SIMPLE headaches, simple relaxation can be effective. Muscle contraction headaches, including common migraines, may respond to easy neck stretches. Move the head to one side and then the other, resisting against the palm of the hand.[143] Tension headaches caused by the neck muscles pulling on the scalp may be helped by chiropractic or craniosacral manipulation.

Aromatherapy is another option. Try rubbing peppermint oil directly on the forehead. Peppermint oil is a natural antispasmodic and diuretic that has been shown in German research to be as effective as Extra Strength Tylenol in easing tension headaches.[144]

The old-fashioned ice pack to the forehead also works; in fact, it has been found to work in about the same amount of time that an analgesic takes to kick in. The ice constricts the swollen blood vessels that cause the head to ache.[145] If an ice pack isn't enough, put the arms in ice water up to the elbows.

Hot compresses can relieve the pain of sinus headaches.

For headaches brought on by stress or tension, a gemmotherapy called Black Currant by Dolisos can help.

Too-low levels of magnesium increase nerve cell excitability and pain.[146] Magnesium supplements have been found to reduce this excitability and migraine susceptibility.

For migraines, the herb feverfew has been touted as a miracle cure that can eliminate the need for drugs. British researchers have found that the herb not only cuts the number and severity of headaches but reduces the nausea that goes with them. Feverfew suppresses the release of prostaglandins and histamines that produce inflammation. In one study, migraine victims who took feverfew capsules for six months were relatively free of migraines, while those taking a placebo suffered three times the normal incidence. In another study, the herb reduced the incidence of migraines by 25 percent and their severity dramatically.[147]

The problem with this herb is that it only works prophylactically. When the drug isn't taken, the headaches return. Homeopathy is a safer remedy that gets to the root of the problem. For migraines, the easiest homeopathic option is a combination remedy by CompliMed called Migramed. The dosage is ten drops three times a day. BHI also makes a combination remedy called Headaches that helps in cases of migraine. Hyland's makes a formula called Headache, which is good for an occasional headache.

Finding the right constitutional homeopathic remedy usually requires consulting a homeopathic physician, who will take a detailed patient history; but you may be able to recognize the symptoms from the following list. The dosage is three pills every fifteen minutes for eight doses. If no relief results, you need a different remedy.

 Homeopathic Options for Tension Headaches

Aconite: for the headache that comes on suddenly; headache after shock or fear, exposure to wind or cold; severe headache during fever

Apis: for head pain behind the left ear, extending to the left eye or temple; the brain feels tired or the head feels swollen; feeling of heat; throbbing pains; better with pressing; worse with motion

Bryonia: left-sided headache; headache over the left eye extending to the occiput, then to the whole head; worse from coughing, in the morning, when constipated, when ironing; better with pressing or with eyes closed

Gelsenium: for the headache beginning at the occiput or neck and radiating to the forehead; worse at ten A.M.; better with urination; head feels very heavy

Ignatia: for the headache that is worse after sweets; headache pain like a nail driven into the head; headache after grief, characterized by sighing

Coffea: for headache resulting from coffee withdrawal, strong stimulation, or strong emotions; headache worse with music, noise, footsteps; headache or migraine pain like a nail driven into the head

Chamomilla: for headache from tooth pain, teething, or earache

Lycopodium: for headache that is worse on the right side, worse from four P.M. to eight P.M. or when trying to concentrate; pain as if temples are being screwed together

Pulsatilla: for headache or migraine that occurs at the end of the menstrual flow; headache that is worse with menopause, heat, sun; worse on exertion or after emotional stress; better with open air, cold applications, pressure; headache pulsates or feels as if it's pressing outward

Silicea: for headache or migraine that begins in occiput and radiates to the forehead or right side of the head; worse from cold, drafts, mental exertion, menstruation, uncovering the head; better when lying with eyes closed or in the dark, or from warming or wrapping the body

Arnica: for headache from trauma or concussion; the head feels bruised or has an aching, sharp pain; worse when stooping

Hypericum: for the bursting, aching headache; worse in damp and fog; headache from contusions or dental work

Nux vomica: for the hangover headache; worse with noise, light, mental activity, before menses; head highly sensitive to stimulation; allergy headache

 ## Homeopathic Options for Migraine Headaches

Iris versicolar: for classic migraine, usually right-sided; pain typically centered in the temple, above or below the eye; vomiting that gives no pain relief; blurred vision preceding headaches; a tight feeling in the scalp

Lac caninum: for headache on alternating sides, either during one attack or from one headache to the next; occipital headache radiating to the forehead

Lac defloratum: for migraine preceded by an aura or dim vision; worse with noise, light, menses; nausea and vomiting present with headache; frontal headache with nausea, vomiting, and chills; headache better with cold applications, lying down, or in the dark

Natrum muriaticum: for the throbbing, blinding headache or migraine that can be felt in any location, often right-sided; "feels like a hammer beating the head"; headache from grief; numbness in face or lips; worse with light, in the sun, when reading, before or after menses, with noise, with head injury, between ten A.M. and three P.M.; better lying in a dark, quiet room; better upon perspiration and with cold applications

Sanguinaria: for the migraine headache that is better after vomiting, with sleep, or after passing gas; migraine on the right side, typically beginning in the neck on the right side and extending to the forehead and eye

HEAD INJURY, UNCONSCIOUSNESS, CONCUSSION

HEAD INJURIES are common in children, whose enthusiasm for running and playing often exceeds their ability to cope with gravity. A loss of consciousness or concussion from a head injury can impair mental function. Children usually feel quiet and subdued for an hour or so after any blow, but if symptoms like vomiting, lethargy, pallor, or an increase in pain are evident, seek the attention of a doctor or emergency room. Symptoms of a serious subdural hemorrhage tend to increase after a period of relative calm. If the child wants to sleep, allow him to do so, but awaken him every twenty minutes or so to assess mental status and offer water. If, after about an hour, the child slips deeper into coma and is hard to rouse, call a pediatrician to check for a subdural hematoma.

 Natural Remedies

THERE ARE several good homeopathic remedies for injuries and trauma. The remedy for head injury is Natrum sulph, usually given in a

high potency. Homeopaths say that anyone who has ever been unconscious needs an initial dose of Nat sulph.

Arnica, the universal remedy for any type of injury, stops the body from overreacting to trauma. Potency varies depending on the seriousness of the injury. Arnica 30c is a good potency to keep around the house for everyday accidents. A more serious accident requires a deeper-acting potency like 200c.

Homeopathic remedies can also release the traumatic impact of past injuries. In one case, a woman who had been knocked unconscious five years earlier complained that she had been unable to smell food cooking since that time. Treatment with Nat sulph brought back her sense of smell. In a second case, a girl who had been knocked unconscious in a car accident was unable to concentrate or study and complained of frequent headaches. Coxsackie series therapy by Staufen relieved these symptoms. Coxsackie is a virus in the spinal column that can travel to the brain when there has been trauma to the head or neck. Comparable series therapy is available in the United States from Deseret.

For other remedies appropriate in specific cases, see a reputable constitutional homeopath.

Goose Egg Shrinks before the Eyes of Amazed Onlookers

A huge welt was beginning to form on the forehead of an accident victim who had collided with the windshield of a car. She was immediately offered Arnica 200c. Two observing doctors watched in amazement as the knot began to shrink within seconds of administration of the dose.

HEAD LICE

HEAD LICE are very small but visible parasites that live in the hair, cause the head to itch, and are highly contagious. The problem is becoming epidemic, striking six million children and adults every year in the United States. A skilled nurse can detect lice feeding on the scalp, but parents may confuse shampoo material with nits hanging on the hair. The definitive symptom is an unignorable scalp itch that is worse at night.

 Conventional Treatment

WHILE THE condition is usually more embarrassing than serious, the drugs used to treat head lice can have serious adverse effects. The usual treatment is shampoos or lotions containing lindane, a chemical poison (formerly sold under the brand name Kwell). This chemical is highly toxic not only to lice but to children; and because it is absorbed through the skin without being neutralized in the stomach, it can go right into the bloodstream. Lindane is a suspected cause of seizures, brain damage, and worse.[148] Kwell's manufacturer stopped making it, but the products are still on store shelves, and generic brands are available and prescribed. Lindane is banned in eighteen countries and severely restricted in ten others. Lindane shampoos are intended for only one or two uses, but many mothers become so frantic over the thought that their children have lice that they go overboard and wash the whole body with it or use it repeatedly.

 Natural Alternatives

A MORE tedious but safer treatment is one that mothers in underdeveloped countries engage in routinely without embarrassment or concern:

they go through the hair every evening with a very fine-toothed comb and systematically remove the nits. Bedding, clothing, hats, and toys should be washed in hot, soapy water to prevent further spread. Everything the child may have touched or laid his head upon should be cleaned either with soap and water or by vacuuming.

A very safe and effective herbal treatment for lice is tea tree oil. Apply the oil directly to the scalp (or on the body for body lice), leave it for about ten minutes, then wash it off. About twenty drops can then be added to half a bottle of shampoo and used in the child's regular hair washings for a week or two afterward.

Tea Tree Oil Works Where Chemical Pesticide Fails

A mother reported using Kwell on her two lice-infested children, yet the lice persisted. She wanted to use the drug again but was advised not to due to its toxicity. Instead, she tried applying tea tree oil, using most of a ten-millileter bottle for her two children and adding the rest to their shampoo. To her relief, the lice completely disappeared.

HEARING IMPAIRMENT, DEAFNESS

HEARING IMPAIRMENT can range from hard of hearing to deafness (although no one seems to be completely deaf). Early detection is important, as language development depends on adequate hearing, and the child may not recognize the problem himself. Never having had normal hearing, he may think his is like everyone else's. If speech is delayed, obtain a screening test. These can be done in infancy but should be administered at least by age four.

Causes of neurosensory hearing loss include rubella and other insults to the fetus during pregnancy, congenital syphilis, hereditary defects, and mumps (though this is rare). If a pregnant woman develops rubella in the first month of her pregnancy, her unborn child has a 50 percent chance of developing an anomaly, and deafness is the most common.

A more common cause of hearing impairment is ear infection, which can cause decreased conductive acuity in the ear. A buildup of fluid in the middle ear prevents sound waves from reaching the nerve that decodes them. This fluid can be removed, but the problem will recur unless the cause of buildup is eliminated. For many children, the underlying problem seems to be a sensitivity to cow's milk, which causes swelling in the ear. In these cases, omitting dairy products from the diet can help. For dietary alternatives, see "Nutrition."

 Conventional Treatment

PARENTS SOMETIMES elect myringotomy (surgical incision of the eardrum, with or without tubes) for children with chronic fluid buildup in the ears, for fear that reduced hearing from the condition will impair learning. But recent research indicates this procedure can do more harm than good and should be reserved only for children who are severely affected. In most cases, chronic fluid buildup eventually clears by itself without surgery, presumably because the skull and eustachian tubes have grown.[149] Antibiotics are routinely prescribed for ear infections, but this practice, too, has been questioned. See "Ear Infections."

For hearing impairment due to wax buildup in the ears, the doctor may mechanically clean the ears with a syringe and water; but this approach isn't very effective, and it can leave fluid in the ears and create other problems. Debrox, an over-the-counter product to remove wax buildup, also leaves fluid in the ears and is not recommended by these authors.

Natural Alternatives

FOR EAR cleaning and to relieve pain from pressure on the eardrum, ear candles are a controversial but effective alternative. The ear candle is a waxed paper cyclinder that is placed in the ear, then burned at the protruding end. The flame creates a vacuum that draws out wax and infection. As a result, fluid moves and the sinuses drain. The FDA hasn't approved ear candles as medical devices, but many people claim remarkable success with their use. Ear candles may improve hearing in addition to relieving pain.

Caution: Not all ear candles are the same. Some can burn too hot, and the wax may melt into the ear, causing burns and other potential damage. Seek professional advice.

For natural relief from ear infections, see "Ear Infections."

HEART MURMURS

A HEART murmur is a swishing sound made by the passage of blood through the chambers of the heart. Most murmurs are innocuous, but certain rare heart lesions that produce murmurs can be fatal. These lesions can usually be surgically corrected. Pediatricians can tell by the location and intensity of the murmur if it is innocuous or requires further investigation. If the child is short of breath, turns blue with exertion, or has other symptoms suggesting compromised circulation, a full pediatric investigation is warranted.

HEAVY-METAL POISONING

HEAVY-METAL ACCUMULATIONS in the brain have been linked to serious neurological disorders, including diseases of older people (Alzheimer's disease, Parkinson's disease, multiple sclerosis) as well as autism in children. The link has been established when victims recovered or improved after the metals were removed from body tissues.[150] Lead poisoning is not the serious problem it once was, since lead has been outlawed in gasoline and is no longer used in paint, but houses built before 1978 still pose a hazard. Children may peel off old lead chips from windowsills and eat them, since they taste sweet. Lead pipes are another source of this toxic heavy metal. Call your local health department if you think your home poses a hazard. If a child is anemic, lethargic, and seems to have headaches, a urine and hair analysis for lead levels can establish a diagnosis of lead poisoning.

 Treatment

HEAVY METALS can be eliminated from the tissues and arteries through chelation. Chelators are substances with extra electrons, or negative charges, that combine with the positive charges of a metal and hold it fast in a clawlike grip. Temperature, acidity, and other environmental changes affect this grip, causing the release and exchange of metals, allowing them to be picked up, transported, and released as needed.

In *Turning Lead into Gold: How Heavy Metal Poisoning Can Affect Your Child and How to Prevent and Treat It* (Vancouver: New Star Books, 1995), Nancy Hallaway, R.N., and Zigurts Strauts, M.D., describe the remarkable reversal of symptoms in several hyperactive, autistic children simply by giving them an oral chelator called Cuprimine (D-penicillamine). Conventional doctors had pronounced the children's conditions hereditary and irreversible, but Dr. Strauts determined that the problem was heavy-metal poisoning resulting from a house remodeling and nearby freeway fumes. (See "Autism.")

EDTA (disodium ethylene diamine tetra-acetic acid) is a chelating substance that has long been used intravenously as a conventional treatment for lead poisoning. Oral chelating drugs are also available, including Cuprimine, DMPS, and DMSA (Chemet).[151] The drugs require a prescription, however, and can result in quite uncomfortable reactions (nausea, vomiting, diarrhea, headache) while toxins are being cleared from the system, particularly in highly toxic people. A gentler approach is to use either natural plant chelators (available in health food stores or supermarkets) or homeopathic chelators.

The chlorophyll in plants is a natural chelator. Cilantro, a leafy green herb, is particularly effective.[152] The problem in the United States is finding a pure source. Cilantro absorbs chemicals so well that most commercial cilantro has absorbed toxins from the air and water. An alternative option more likely to be uncontaminated is the freshwater algae chlorella. The recommended dose is ½ teaspoon a day, up to 1½ teaspoons according to tolerance.

Alpha-lipoic acid is a very powerful antioxidant that can bind to toxic metals, increasing the liver's detoxification and metabolic enzyme production abilities. It is both water- and fat-soluble, so it can travel to and permeate all the cells of the body, including the brain. ALA is present naturally in spinach, kidney, heart, skeletal muscle (beef), and broccoli, and can be purchased in concentrated form as a supplement.[153]

Homeopathic chelators are also available. Their effectiveness was demonstrated in a laboratory study in which rats were given crude doses of arsenic, bismuth, cadmium, mercury chloride, or lead. Animals pretreated with homeopathic doses of these substances before and after exposure to the crude substances excreted more of the toxic crude substances through urine, feces, and sweat than did animals pretreated with a placebo.[154]

A new line of combination homeopathic products has been designed specifically for neutralizing heavy-metal poisoning, dental work, and environmental toxins. Oratox by Deseret should be used for two or three weeks after dental work. Other Deseret combination homeopathics include Enviroclenz and Metox. A remedy by PCHF (Professional Complementary Health Formulas) called Amalgam is particularly good for clearing mercury amalgam from body tissues. Other options are Amalgam by PHP and Protomer by Futureplex. Supplemental zinc is good to help counteract mercury and nickel absorption.

To neutralize the harmful effects of dental and other X rays, give Radiation Drops by Deseret, once before and three times after the X ray. Molecular Biologicals makes homeopathic drops by the same name.

Heavy-metal Poisoning from Licking Paintbrushes Relieved

A young man who had begun oil painting at the age of eleven complained of chronic fatigue syndrome, tiredness, sudden drops in energy, frequent colds, flus, and increasingly frequent attacks of environmental sensitivities. He was strongly affected by the smell of perfume, paint, or chemicals. A review of his history revealed that his health had begun deteriorating several years after he began oil painting. He recalled habitually sticking the brushes in his mouth after soaking them with paint, to help form the proper brush stroke. Hair analysis showed many toxic metals in his body, including high levels of cobalt, mercury, manganese, and copper. Homeopathic metal detox drops stopped his attacks of environmental sensitivity and improved his overall health.

HEPATITIS

HEPATITIS IS an inflammation of the liver caused by a virus and characterized by a dull, constant ache or fullness in the liver area, usually accompanied by jaundice. Jaundice shows as a yellow tint to the whites of the eyes and in severe cases to the skin, resulting when toxins accumulate in the blood. (See "Jaundice.")

Two types of hepatitis are common. Infectious hepatitis (type A) is transferred from person to person, usually by mouth; serum hepatitis (type B) is passed in the blood. Hepatitis B can be passed from mother to child or through sexual contact, blood transfusions, or the shared needles of intravenous-drug users. Most victims recover completely, but some develop chronic hepatitis and possibly cirrhosis of the liver. Hepatitis A, the least dangerous form of hepatitis, does not cause long-term liver damage. It is usually transmitted through food or water from fecal matter (for example, from restaurant workers who don't wash their hands). Symptoms include loss of appetite, fatigue, mild fever, muscle or joint aches, nausea, vomiting, abdominal pain, dark urine, and jaundice. Hepatitis A takes about a month after exposure to manifest symptoms. The contagious period is about two weeks preceding the height of the illness (fever, jaundice, tender liver—the abdominal area below the last rib on the right side of the body). Children are usually allowed to return to school three weeks after the onset of symptoms. They may be out of sorts for a month afterward.

 ## Conventional Treatment

CONVENTIONAL MEDICINE has little to offer for hepatitis. Certain drugs have been tried experimentally, but none are clearly effective. Hepatitis B vaccines are available, and many health authorities are now recommending them for newborns; but contracting the disease is likely only for prostitutes, homosexuals, and intravenous-drug users, and the vaccines are so controversial that doctors themselves often refuse to take them.

 ## The Alternative Approach

GERMAN HOMEOPATHIC remedies by Staufen called Hepatitis A and Hepatitis B are highly effective alternatives. They are available in the United States as series therapy from Deseret.

Herbal supplements useful for cleaning the liver include milk thistle and yellow dock. Vitamin C and the herb silymarin can also help relieve symptoms. Adequate rest and a good diet are important for recovery.

The conventional view is that diet has nothing to do with hepatitis, and that the patient can eat whatever he wants. But alternative practitioners maintain that proper diet is key to clearing any liver disease from the system. The liver's chief function is to detoxify the body. Besides the harmful by-products of metabolism, it has to deal with pesticides, pollutants, drugs, and toxic chemicals. A diet emphasizing greens can clean the liver and reduce recovery time dramatically. The liver needs to be given a rest from proteins, which are hard for it to handle and should be eaten only in very small amounts, if at all. The Liver Cleanse Diet is described in detail under "Environmental Illness."

HERNIA

AN *INGUINAL hernia* is a weakness in the muscular abdominal wall that allows a loop of small bowel to protrude. These hernias are more common in males, since the opening that allows the sperm duct from the testes to pass through to the urethra may be subject to extrusion. The pediatrician will detect a swelling that feels like a little balloon just to the left or right of the pubic bone. The hernia can usually be pushed back into place, but with coughing or straining, it will protrude again. A device called a truss can be used but is not curative; surgery is generally required. Anesthesia for this surgery is usually light, as the abdomen does not have to be entered. Occasionally the hernia will come out and push its way down into the scrotum, where it can twist and become incarcerated. In that case, an emergency operation is necessary.

An *umbilical hernia* is a defect in the abdominal wall noted shortly after birth, resulting when the skin around the navel does not close after the vessels in the cord have dried up and fallen off. This defect has nothing to do with the way the obstetrician has tied the cord. It usually resolves on its own, but surgery is sometimes required. The protrusion is normally taped flat, although the tape can cause a rash.

HICCUPS

HICCUPS ARE intermittent spasms of the diaphragm muscle precipitated by a full stomach or some irritating food in the stomach. Among other home remedies, taking sips of cold water or a spoonful of dry sugar may help.

If hiccups persist, a homeopathic remedy by Dolisos called Hiccups is reported to be effective. Another homeopathic combination approach includes the remedies Cuprum metallicum 9c and Hyoscyamus niger 9c. Alternate three pellets of each remedy every two minutes until hiccups stop. If they occur from overeating, use Nux vomica 6c or 30x.

HIGH BLOOD PRESSURE
(See Hypertension)

HIP DYSPLASIA

CONGENITAL DISLOCATION of the hip results when the head of the femur (thigh bone) does not sit correctly in the pelvis. If treatment isn't undertaken at an early age, ambulation will be poor or clumsy later, but the condition is sometimes overlooked if the doctor does not examine for it. The femur will then slide up the side of the pelvic bone when the child starts to walk. At that advanced age, the condition is difficult to treat, so testing for it should be done in the newborn. This is accomplished by maneuvering the femur in different positions to check for stability. If the femur does not fit into its joint space, the condition will sometimes show as more folds in the skin of the affected side. A clicking sound may also be heard on manipulation. The condition is confirmed by X ray.

 ## Conventional Treatment

CURRENT THERAPY is a cast to keep the leg in an abducted (spread-eagle) position so a space for the femur head can be established. The treatment takes months, however, and can be traumatic for the child.

 ## Natural Alternatives

DIFFERENT TYPES of manual manipulation, including craniosacral therapy and a form of bodywork called Zero Balancing, have been reported effective in correcting congenital hip dislocation and other structural irregularities due to genetics or a traumatic birth. For further information on Zero Balancing, call 831-476-0665 or see the website www.zerobalancing.com. For a craniosacral therapist in your area, call the Cranial Academy in Indianapolis at 317-594-0411, or check the website of the Upledger Institute, www.upledger.com.

Hip Dysplasia Cured with Zero Balancing Technique

A boy with a type of hip dysplasia called Perthe's disease was put into a full-length cast at the age of five. When the cast was removed, he could not walk without crutches. His father, an orthopedic surgeon, elected to try Zero Balancing. The boy received weekly treatments over a period of several years. At the age of eight, he is now crutches-free and Rollerblading.

HIVES (See Itching)

HYPERACTIVITY (See ADD)

HYPERTENSION (HIGH BLOOD PRESSURE)

HYPERTENSION IS rare in children, but blood pressure is routinely checked by pediatricians just in case. If there is a rise in blood pressure, the usual cause is a kidney or heart condition or obesity. A definitive diagnosis must be made by the doctor, then the underlying condition is treated.

HYPOGLYCEMIA

HYPOGLYCEMIA (LOW blood sugar) is the flip side of diabetes (high blood sugar). Hypoglycemia usually results from the ingestion of sugary foods, although foods to which a person is sensitive can sometimes cause it. Eating sugary foods causes the body to secrete large amounts of insulin. In the hypoglycemic person, the sugar is used up before the insulin, causing the blood sugar to drop too low.

Blood sugar rises sharply after a high-carbohydrate meal, stimulating the release of insulin to push the sugar into cells or to store it as fat. Blood sugar then suddenly drops, creating an alarm reaction in the body. Low blood sugar can set stress hormones racing. When adrenaline is released, the same physiological symptoms result as if the child had seen an approaching bear: anxiety, sweaty palms, a feeling of impending doom and of the need to hide or run. The ability to concentrate also diminishes. If the child is in school, an erroneous diagnosis may be made of ADD (see ADD). If the syndrome occurs in the middle of the night after ice cream or other sugary foods at bedtime, the child may awaken with thrashing, screaming, a rapid heartbeat, and dilated pupils. (See "Night Terrors.")

 Natural Remedies

THE RECOMMENDED treatment is to eat a complex carbohydrate food or a protein snack every three hours. Eliminate sugar sources, and serve protein with every meal: Almonds are particularly good. Hypoglycemia is corrected by the same natural blood sugar balancers as is diabetes. Chromium picolinate taken with lunch and dinner can help balance out the blood sugar. (See "Diabetes.") High-dose vitamin C (about 1,000 to 3,000 milligrams daily), along with pantothenic acid, can help restore mental and physical equilibrium by bolstering the functioning of the adrenal glands.

HYPOTHYROIDISM, HYPERTHYROIDISM

HYPOTHYROIDISM IS the deficient production of thyroid hormone. The congenital form is rare but should not be missed, since delayed treatment can retard mental development, and treatment is simple and cheap. The affected infant may show lethargy, excessively long periods of sleep, slow growth, cold skin, and a yellow pallor. X rays of the wrist bones can detect delayed osseous (bone) development, and a blood test can detect insufficient thyroid hormone.

Hyperthyroidism, or an excess of thyroid hormone, is most commonly seen in a condition called Graves' disease. Symptoms include nervousness, irritability, sweating, and muscle weakness.

Postpartum thyroiditis is an overactivity of the thyroid gland occurring in a mother a few months after childbirth. The condition may be followed by underactivity of the thyroid a few weeks later.

Drug Treatment

THE USUAL medication for an underactive thyroid is synthetic thyroxine (levothyroxine or Synthroid). Once the patient begins taking it, however, he or she is liable to be on it for life. Another drawback is that the same stress that blocks the thyroid can block conversion of the synthetic hormone to T3 (triiodothyronine), the form in which thyroid hormone is most active in the body.[155] There may also be side effects, including heart palpitations, insomnia, nervousness, and diarrhea. If thyroid therapy is necessary, it should be prescribed by a competent professional. Excess thyroid supplementation may be harmful, since it stimulates the osteoclasts, the cells that tear down or resorb bone.[156]

Conventional treatment for Graves' disease consists of antithyroid drugs that cause hormone production to drop—methimazole (Tapazole) or propylthiouracil (PTU). If the drugs fail, a high-dose radioactive iodine capsule or beverage is given that slows the thyroid by permanently damaging overactive cells. But if too many cells are destroyed (as is often the case), the patient winds up on hormone supplements for life.[157]

Some doctors prescribe drugs to relieve the anxiety and nervousness of postpartum thyroiditis, but the underlying condition generally goes away by itself.

Natural Alternatives

FOR HYPOTHYROIDISM, a more natural and less habit-forming option is Armour Thyroid, a desiccated thyroid preparation extracted from pigs. Like Synthroid, Armour Thyroid is standardized to government specifications to allow proper monitoring.

Acupuncture can also help stimulate thyroid function, and supplementing with trace minerals may help. Thyroid function is dependent on a balance of two trace minerals, manganese and iodine: Hypothyroidism could be due to a shortage of either.

Herbal thyroid stimulants include dulse and kelp, both high in iodine. People who ingest large quantities of soy products need extra iodine, since daily soy taken in quantity can suppress the thyroid. The Asian diet, which is high in soy, is also high in kelp and seaweed.

Homeopathic remedies that work to correct the problem at its source are also available. Homeopathy regulates the thyroid gland so the body can function normally without drugs.

Hyperthyroidism can be a function of the same hormonal imbalance that produces an underactive thyroid. These cases need to be evaluated by a medical doctor, but homeopathic remedies can help rebalance the system. See a constitutional homeopath.

Lifetime Thyroid Drug Dependency Avoided

Kara had been diagnosed as hypothyroid at the age of sixteen and had been on Synthroid for nearly a decade. Her doctor said she would have to take the drug for life; but after nine years of this course of treatment, she asked to switch to Armour Thyroid, and her doctor reluctantly agreed. After about three months on Armour Thyroid, Kara began taking homeopathic Thyroid by CompliMed. Throughout this treatment, lab tests showed her thyroid levels to be normal. In the last four years, she has taken just the Thyroid homeopathic, and that only three times, for a month each time. For the past eight months, she has needed nothing in the way of supplements, and her thyroid function has remained normal.

IMMUNITY

COLDS, FLUS, and ear infections are endemic among children, who are exposed at school to everything that is going around. As a result, they often wind up on repeated courses of antibiotics, but these drugs are losing their effectiveness. An increasing incidence of staph infections and otitis media (middle-ear infection) among children is blamed on the overuse of broad-spectrum microbial drugs.[158] Not only are antibiotics becoming ineffective, but they depress the immunological response to bacteria, preventing the development of natural antibodies and interfering with the development of natural immunity; and they permit overgrowths by resistant Candida microbes, which then produce toxins that can weaken the immune system and further reduce resistance.[159] Immune-suppressing steroids like cortisone give infections even greater opportunity to spread (see "Itching"). Alternative practitioners argue that common childhood infections should be allowed to run their course without drug intervention, since they are necessary for building a strong immune system and represent a natural cleansing process that eliminates toxins. Meanwhile, safe and effective natural immune boosters and pain relievers are available to relieve symptoms.

 Drug Treatment

ANTIBIOTICS ARE the conventional answer to bacterial infection, but bacteria have had more than half a century to adapt and become resistant. Predictions are that in a few more years, antibiotics won't be available to treat the serious diseases for which these medicines have earned their reputation as lifesaving wonder drugs.

Antibiotic resistance is attributed to overuse of the drugs in both animals and humans. Well over a million antibiotic prescriptions are written yearly for colds; yet *colds are caused by viruses, and antibiotics have no effect against these marauders*. The professed justification is prophylactic: to treat any bacterial infection that *might* arise. The problems with this theory are that if an infection does develop, the bacteria will have had an opportunity to become resistant to the antibiotic; and the patient runs the unnecessary risk of developing an allergic reaction to the drug.

Antibiotic resistance is also blamed on the livestock industry, which purchases an astounding half of all antibiotics sold. The drugs are incorporated into feed to kill bacteria that stunt the growth of the animals. Resistant bacteria then develop and multiply, and when humans eat the animals, they can become infected with the resistant strains. Cooking the meat will kill the bacteria, but the antibiotic remains in the flesh and is absorbed into the bloodstream after ingestion of the meat. Milk products are also laced with antibiotics. The doses absorbed are low but are sufficient to allow the bacteria to develop a resistance to the drug. Another suspected source of antibiotic resistance is the use of antibacterial soaps in the kitchen, which give the organisms an opportunity to adapt to the soap's antibacterial agents.

 Natural Immune System Boosters

CHILD LIFE, a new company based in Los Angeles, has a variety of good natural products for building immunity. One called First Defense is designed to boost the immune system at the first sign of a cold or flu. It includes a long list of immune boosters, including olive-leaf extract, a natural antibiotic and antiviral shown to be useful against a wide range of diseases.[160]

Elderberry extract (Sambucus nigra) is another popular herbal remedy for colds and flu that comes in chewable flavors for children. Rather than merely suppressing the body's eliminatory mechanisms, elderberry extract has been shown to actually halt the spread of infection. A recent study suggests that it can significantly reduce the length and severity of flu symptoms.[161] In an Israeli study, an extract of the herb cut flu recovery times in half.[162]

Echinacea is another herb that helps strengthen the immune system's ability to ward off pathogens. It is a good product to boost your child's immune system when other children are sick, or if your child has frequent colds or recurring ear infections. It should not be used, however, when a cold is in full force (see "Colds"). Child Life makes an orange-flavored liquid Echinacea for preschool and school-aged children. The same company makes a good-tasting liquid multivitamin/multimineral supplement that helps support the immune system.

Herbs for Kids also makes a line of children's products for boosting the immune system, including Astragalus, Echinacea/Astragalus, and Echinacea/Goldenseal in blackberry and orange flavors. All are alcohol-free.

A cell salt called Bioplasma is an immune system booster popular with children. Cell salts are low-potency homeopathic remedies made from naturally occurring salt minerals that make up the body's structure. Bioplasma is easy to swallow, tastes like candy, and dissolves easily. The recommended dose is four pills three times a day. Also good for boosting the immune system of the child with chronic colds is the cell salt Ferrum phos in a 6x potency three to four times daily. Thymactive by NF Formulas is a homeopathic product good for strengthening the immune system, available as liquid drops or tablets.

Colostrum is another effective immune-booster. Derived from the first milk of cows, it is now available in pill form. In many reported cases, taking colostrum capsules every hour or two at the first sign of a cold has kept the cold from developing.

Vitamin C and the trace mineral zinc are well known for their ability to reduce the duration and severity of colds. For research and dosages, see "Colds."

To speed recovery from infection, try the warm-socks treatment. Soak the child's feet in a hot bath for ten minutes, then wet a pair of cotton socks with cold water. Wring them out, put them on the child's feet, and immediately cover with a pair of dry wool socks. Then put the child to bed. The wet socks are uncomfortable for only a minute. By morning, the body will have heated and dried the socks; and the immune system, circulation, and white blood count all will have gotten a boost in the process.

A time-honored remedy for a weak immune system is ultraviolet light from the sun. In the nineteenth century, frail or sickly children were sent to the beach for the summer to recuperate. Sunbathing and UV therapy were considered the most effective treatments for many infectious diseases, including tuberculosis, until penicillin was discovered in 1938. Sun therapy was then forgotten, as drugs became big business.[163] But now nature herself is forcing us to return to her own remedies, including prudent sunbathing. (See "Sunburn.")

IMMUNIZATIONS

CHILDHOOD IMMUNIZATION is considered so important that parents who refuse to vaccinate their children, even for religious reasons, have been held subject to charges of child abuse. As with most drugs, however, there are two sides to the issue. Immunizations are based on the theory that immunity to the usual childhood diseases can be induced by injecting a small amount of the offending germ into the child. But so many vaccines have been added to the prescribed regimen that they represent a huge load on the immature immune system, with the potential for long-term side effects; and some children still get the diseases the shots were designed to prevent.

The vaccine schedule suggested by the American Academy of Pediatrics is as follows: Hepatitis B on the first day of life and again at two months and twelve months; DPT (diphtheria/pertussis/tetanus) at two, four, and six months; polio at two, four, and six months (first by injection, then oral drops), with a polio oral booster at five years; boosters of DPT at eighteen months and five years; hemophilus influenza bacteria (Hib) at two months, four months, six months, and again in the next few months; and MMR (measles/mumps/rubella) at fifteen months, with a booster at age five. Chicken pox vaccine has also been added to the list, as well as a Td booster at about fifteen years (diphtheria/tetanus without the pertussis of the earlier DPT shot).

Vaccine Hazards

IMMUNIZATIONS CAN produce side effects ranging from mild fever and sore muscles to severe screaming, high fever, and death. Vaccines have been linked to sudden infant death syndrome (SIDS), autism, and certain autoimmune diseases, including hypothyroidism, allergies, and multiple sclerosis. While the official position is that complications from vaccines are rare, the counterargument is that complications may simply not be reported, since they can show up long after the vaccines were administered and are hard to trace. Moreover, reactions that were rare when the studies were first done may not be rare today, because infants are second- or third-generation vaccine recipients with potentially heightened reactions when rechallenged with the vaccine.

SIDS has been linked to the DPT vaccine (given at two, four, and six months) and the hepatitis B vaccine (given at two months). The Vaccine Adverse Event Reporting System contains about 25,000 reports of adverse reactions associated with the hepatitis B vaccine, including 440 deaths. The findings include brain edema in healthy infants who die very soon after receiving the vaccine.[164] The MMR vaccine, which is given at fifteen months, has been linked to autism, a condition that generally appears at about eighteen months. There are now a minimum of 250,000 autistic children in the United States, a ten- to fifteen-fold increase since immunization came into vogue. Dr. Bernard Rimland, founding director of the Autism Research Institute, blames childhood-vaccine programs. Childhood autism is caused by encephalitis (brain inflammation) affecting the limbic system of the brain. The MMR is first incubated in chick embryo culture. The concern is that the virus becomes programmed to produce antibodies against the protein of the myelin sheath of the chick and then of the child.[165]

Less obvious consequences of vaccines involve the immune system. Symptoms of the most common communicable diseases for which vaccines are given (measles, rubella, mumps, chicken pox) are usually mild, and contracting these diseases once generally affords immunity for life. Several studies have linked autoimmune diseases, including allergies, asthma, and diabetes, to immunization and a decreased incidence of childhood infections. These autoimmune diseases are rare in parts of the world, in parts of town, and in families where childhood diseases are allowed to run their course, giving the immune system something to "cut its teeth" on. In a 1997 study of nearly three hundred children in Guinea-Bissau, allergies (asthma, eczema, hay fever, etc.) were found to be significantly more common in children who had *not* had measles. Vaccination evidently did not give the same protection as the disease itself. Other recent studies suggest that exposure to hepatitis A, tuberculosis, and other infections helps build immunity to allergies. The suggested explanation is that the evolving immune system needs to keep busy. If it has no invaders to cope with, it turns its defenses on otherwise harmless stimuli.[166]

Also in dispute is whether the decline in the major childhood killers in the first half of the twentieth century can actually be credited to vaccines. With the exception of polio, the incidence of those diseases had already dropped by 95 percent before mass vaccine programs were instituted. This decline is attributed to better housing with less crowded conditions after the Depression, better nutrition, and better public health measures.[167] As for polio, one researcher has shown that its rise and fall directly paralleled the widespread use and withdrawal from the market of DDT and other pesticides that are highly toxic to the nervous system. This correlation, he maintains, could explain the rise and fall in incidence of the disease rather than use of the vaccine.[168]

 ## Natural Therapies

SOME PARENTS choose to allow their children to develop permanent immunity to common childhood diseases like measles and chicken pox from the diseases themselves. Although this option, too, poses risks, they are remote. German measles carries a risk of brain inflammation, which could cause degeneration; but the chance is only $\frac{1}{10}$ of 1 percent. Parents need to do some research and weigh the risks themselves. If they choose to forego immunizations, a good diet, extra vitamin C, and certain homeopathic remedies can minimize discomfort and risks for the child. Homeopathic remedies work on the same principle as vaccines: They innoculate the body with a tiny bit of the toxin, stimulating the production of antibodies that fight the disease. The advantage of homeopathy is that so little of the original toxin is left in the remedy that the patient cannot accidently contract the disease or be burdened with its latent toxic effects. Homeopathic remedies by the German company Staufen are available for each of the childhood communicable diseases; Deseret series therapy is the American version of these remedies.

Parents who choose immunization are cautioned not to allow their children to be vaccinated when sick. The child should be in full health, with no runny nose, fever, or other symptoms. Pediatricians sometimes say these symptoms are unimportant to the vaccine process, but alternative health care professionals feel strongly that they increase the risk of side effects.

If vaccines are elected, homeopathic remedies can help prevent side effects if taken before and after the injections. Thuja helps keep the body from overreacting to the drugs. Three tablets given in a 6x or 30x dosage before and after the injection aid the body in recovering quickly. Give a few extra doses (three pills daily for three days) if the child has a fever or rash from the immunization. A higher dosage (200c or 1m) of this remedy may be given by a homeopath who finds problems from immunizations months or years afterward.

Thuja is also the appropriate remedy for an allergic reaction to vaccines. Silicea is another option. Some homeopaths give homeopathic sulphur to a child who gets red and swollen at the site of an injection or who appears to be going into shock. CompliMed makes a remedy called Vaccinations that is good for relieving the effects of a previously administered vaccine. For anaphylactic shock from vaccines, see "Shock."

**Lingering Vaccine Symptoms
Relieved with Natural Remedy**

Thirty-two-year-old Debbie said she had never been well since she had received a series of tuberculosis injections to test for the disease. In the test, a small amount of the TB virus is injected under the skin; a doctor or nurse then checks a few days later to see if there is a reaction. Debbie had a strong feeling that this test was the beginning of her detoriorating health. A dose of Tuberculinum recommended by a homeopath cleared a number of health problems along with her complaints of lowered immunity.

IMPETIGO

IMPETIGO IS a bacterial skin infection that can develop from scraped skin or a cut. Children like to pick at sores. The result can be to inoculate the sore with either a strep or staph bacillus. In the extreme case, the infection can cause heart or kidney complications, but this result is very rare.

Drug Treatment

ANTIBIOTIC OINTMENTS like Neosporin are sometimes used, but they can sensitize the skin and actually worsen the condition. Widespread impetigo may be treated with a systemic oral antibiotic. For downsides, see "Itching."

Natural Alternatives

HOME CARE includes daily bathing of sores with soap and water, then applying a clean, dry dressing. This may be all that is needed, but a natural healing ointment like Calendula and Hypericum cream may also be applied. Hypericum eliminates nerve pain.

European Walnut, a gemmotherapy made by Dolisos, is a good herbal remedy for staph/strep skin eruptions: It heals the skin by clearing toxins from the system. It is taken in water, ten to fifty drops in a single daily dose.

Homeopathic remedies can also speed recovery. Bacticin drops by CompliMed boost the immune system to clear infections. Give children five drops three times daily. Deseret makes a product called Staph/Strep specifically to fight staph and strep infections.

The homeopathic formula Thymactive by NF Formulas can help the body fight off infection. Certain herbs and nutrients can also give an overall boost to the immune system, including colostrum, goldenseal, and echinacea. Colloidal silver is another possibility. (See "Immunity.")

INDIGESTION (See Stomachache)

INFANT FEEDING (See Nutrition)

INFECTION (See Immunity, Colds)

INFLAMMATION (See Pain)

INFLUENZA (See Flu)

INJURIES (See Trauma)

INSECT BITES AND STINGS

INSECT BITES can annoy and lead to infection, since children tend to scratch them until they bleed. However, insect repellants may represent a more serious risk to children than the bites themselves. Excessive or prolonged use of ordinary repellants has caused serious reactions in infants and young children, and only brief exposure to small amounts of the higher-concentration products has caused serious reactions in both children and adults, including anaphylactic shock and grand mal seizures. Swallowing DEET (N,N-diethyl-m-toluamide), the active ingredient in most popular brands, can be fatal.

Insect bites can also be fatal, but no drugstore repellants are effective against the most dangerous of the biting insects, the stinging Hymenoptera. This insect family, which includes bees, wasps, hornets, yellow jackets, and fire ants, is collectively responsible for more deaths each year in the United States than any other poisonous animals, including rattlesnakes.

Normal reactions to insect stings include pain, redness, swelling, itching, and warmth at the site of the bite. These reactions can be quite painful, but so long as they're confined to the area of the sting, they're considered normal inflammatory responses. The reactions that require emergency treatment are those from multiple bites, which can produce toxic reactions in normal children; and in sensitive children, allergic reactions to a single bite can be just as serious. **When determining whether to call a doctor if your child is stung, look for these symptoms: severe pain, redness or itching at the site of the sting; sudden, serious swelling of the lips, tongue, eyes, or body; itching all over the body; hives (itchy bumps on the skin); wheezing, sudden coughing, or trouble breathing; dizziness and weakness; serious nausea; or collapse.**

Conventional Treatment and Prevention

DRUGS USED to treat serious allergic reactions to insect bites include epinephrine by injection, antihistamines by injection or mouth, and adrenal steroids. If you know your child is allergic to insect stings, keep an emergency insect-treatment kit on hand that contains these items (available by prescription).

For prevention, topical insect repellants are sold at drugstores and supermarkets. Most biting insects, including mosquitoes, chiggers, ticks, and biting flies, can be driven off by these products; but again, they don't work on the stinging Hymenoptera. DEET, the active ingredient in Off and most other popular brands, can cause a variety of health problems, from dizziness to death. In 1995, 6,745 DEET poisonings were reported to the American Association of Poison Control Centers, including 4,332 for children under six and one fatality in an adult. Numerous cases of DEET-related problems are also thought to go unreported. Many people are not aware that chemicals sprayed on the skin are absorbed into the circulation. About 10 to 15 percent of each dose of DEET can be recovered from the urine.

Natural Alternatives

THESE RISKS can be avoided by using a nontoxic insect repellant. Formulated from all-natural plant oils, these products are quite effective.

Buzz Away by Quantum contains citronella oil, eucalyptus, lemongrass, cedarwood, and peppermint oils. It has passed EPA safety and efficacy tests and is rated effective against mosquitoes for two and a half hours after application. Green Ban is another effective DEET-free repellant.

A homeopathic remedy called Biting Insects by Molecular Biologicals discourages insects remarkably well if taken orally a few hours before exposure.

An insect repellant popular among campers is Avon's Skin-So-Soft, a concentrated bath oil. In one study, Skin-So-Soft successfully repelled the mosquito that carries yellow fever. The *Medical Letter* cautions, however, that this remedy may be effective for as little as ten to thirty minutes, compared to one to several hours for products containing DEET.

Another natural insect repellant is the B vitamin thiamin (B_1) taken orally. (Brewer's yeast tablets also work, but you may have trouble getting your child to swallow them.) Vitamin B_1 works best if used daily for at least a week before it is needed. It will then be detectable through the pores of the skin by bugs, which are repelled by the smell. Recommended dosages are 100 milligrams per day for adults and children over ten years of age, and 50 milligrams per day for children under ten years of age. Don't use on children under three. Adding large portions of onions and garlic to the diet can discourage insects from biting through the same mechanism.

If your child gets stung by a bee, you can reduce inflammation by licking an aspirin and applying it to the bite. Also good for treating insect bites is homeopathic Apis 6x or 30x (three pills every fifteen minutes for one hour); Dolisos makes an Apis cream. Calendula cream is another safe treatment for bites. Avoid antibiotic creams, which can cause sensitization of the skin among other side effects (see "Itching").

To reduce the likelihood of bites, dress children in close-fitting clothes that cover as much of the body as possible and won't attract insects. Brightly colored clothes may be mistaken for flowers, but dark-colored clothing (brown or black) may also provoke an attack. The least interesting materials to bees are white or light khaki. Scented soaps, perfumes, suntan lotions and other cosmetics, and shiny jewelry or buckles can also attract stinging insects.[169]

Bees won't attack unless their hives are threatened or they are stepped on. After a sting, remove the stinger and attached venom sac, since these can continue to inject venom after being torn from the insect. Ice can help lessen pain and swelling.

Bee Sting Relieved with Homeopathic Remedy

Author Dr. Walker's four-year-old nephew was playing in the pool when he suddenly began screaming and crying uncontrollably, having been stung by a bee. Dr. Walker got homeopathic Apis from her kit and tried to give it to the boy, but he was crying too hard to take it. She then put a few pellets of Apis 30c on his tongue. The minute it touched his mouth, he stopped crying; and within two minutes, he was back in the pool playing and having fun. Not another word was heard about the sting, and there was no swelling, redness, or pain.

INSOMNIA, SLEEP DISORDERS

ONE OF the major challenges and triumphs of parenthood is getting children to sleep through the night. In infancy, they awaken every couple of hours to nurse. The transition to adult sleeping habits takes a number of years. In the meantime, parents have to adjust their own sleeping patterns, a stressful proposition when they have adult daytime schedules to maintain.

Besides the normal incompatibility between children's and adults' sleeping patterns, a number of stressors can cause wakefulness in children. They include earaches and other pains, allergies, stress, anxiety, depression, travel and other changes in routine, being overtired, fits of temperament, colas and other caffeinated drinks, and chocolate. Insomnia can also be caused by drugs containing stimulants, including over-the-counter nasal decongestants, asthma products, and diet aids; painkillers like Anacin and Excedrin, which contain caffeine; and many prescription drugs, including those for asthma, coughs, and colds.

Sleep is a habit that is encouraged by a regular bedtime ritual (the bath, bedtime story, prayers) at the same time each night. Stimulating video games, television programs, physically active games, running and other heavy exercise should be discouraged near bedtime. A good practice is to devote ten minutes of "talk time" to each of your children each night. This is a time for bonding one-on-one, when problems can be discussed and the child can be assured of your undivided attention.

 ## Drug Treatment

DOCTORS SOMETIMES suggest drugs for children's sleeping problems, most commonly antihistamines like Benadryl. Stronger drugs are also occasionally prescribed for childhood insomnia, including benzodiazepines (Valium, Xanax) and sedatives or barbiturates.[170] These drugs can make the child drowsy and "hungover" the next day, and some can have more serious side effects. Barbiturates and benzodiazepines, which are available only by prescription, can depress brain function, be addictive, and cause crises on withdrawal.

 ## Natural Alternatives

BACH FLOWER and homeopathic remedies are effective sleep aids that have absolutely no side effects. Rescue Remedy is a popular Bach flower combination that can bring on the relaxation required to fall asleep. It is particularly effective for children after a stressful day.

Chamomile is an excellent homeopathic remedy for inducing sleep in restless children. Another is Passiflora 3x or 6x. The recommended dosage is two pills twenty minutes after dinner, two before bed, and two if waking occurs in the night. Users report that in a few days, sleep continues through the night and results in waking refreshed, not drowsy. This ritual also helps to reset erratic sleep patterns. There are also many effective combination homeopathic remedies for insomnia, including Quietiva by CompliMed and Quietude by Boiron.

Homeopathic Melatonin 12x is appropriate for children whose time clock is off, either from jet lag or in cases where they're staying up late and sleeping well into the next day. It works by stimulating the body to produce its own melatonin, a hormone secreted by the pineal gland when darkness falls. Although nonhomeopathic melatonin is not recommended for children, for parents (especially fathers) having trouble falling asleep after being awakened by a restless child, melatonin in capsule form can be quite effective.

Aromatherapy is also calming and relaxing. Try lavender oil in the bedroom, by or on the child's pillow or on a rag placed near the bed, or burn a lavender-scented candle in the room. Pillows are also made with lavender seeds in them. Chamomile oil is good for the child who has trouble relaxing or is hyperactive, nervous, or upset.

Among nutrients, the amino acid L-tryptophan is an effective sleep inducer for both adults and children. It was removed from the market in 1989 after several deaths occurred from its use, but the deaths were later traced to a single contaminated batch from Japan rather than to L-tryptophan itself. For children, a safe source of this amino acid is milk (breast or cow), a time-honored bedtime food. Turkey and pumpkin seeds are other options.

The traditional hot drink, bedtime story, and hot bath are other time-tested aids to sleep. Teas containing a combination of relaxing herbs for bedtime are on the market. Herbs that can help induce sound sleep include chamomile, valerian, passionflower, and skullcap. For children, honey and milk can improve the appeal, although honey should not be given to children under one year old. (See "Nutrition.")

Another bedtime ritual was suggested by Dr. John R. Christopher, a renowned herbalist. He maintains that static electricity that has built up in the body—exaggerated by wearing rubber-soled shoes—prevents people from getting a good night's sleep. To counter it, he recommends a barefoot walk in the grass before bed.

For the child who awakens in the middle of the night, suspect pinworms or hypoglycemia. See "Parasites," "Hypogylcemia," "Night Terrors."

INTESTINAL FLU

INTESTINAL FLU is a viral infection of the intestinal tract. In children, it runs a predictable course. The typical intestinal flu starts with a low-grade fever (99 to 101 degrees Fahrenheit) and vomiting for twenty-four hours, followed by a week of watery diarrhea with cramps. Many children get this flu once every year or two (when it "goes around"). Each time they get it, it lasts a day or so less due to a developed immunity. Most adults have it for only one day.

 Treatment

SINCE INTESTINAL flu is caused by a virus, antibiotics won't work on it. (See "Immunity.") The condition will generally pass of its own accord, but it is important that the child get enough fluids to prevent dehydration. If urination occurs at least twice a day, fluid intake is probably sufficient.

Sucking on ice chips helps relieve nausea. When vomiting stops and the main complaint is watery diarrhea, fluids may be given by mouth. Also try soda crackers, bananas, applesauce, and gelatin. The low-roughage BRAT diet is routinely recommended: bananas, rice, applesauce, and toast.

The first-choice homeopathic remedy for children's stomach cramps, particularly from intestinal flu, is Arsenicum alba. Give it in a low potency (6x, 6c, 30x, or 30c) at a dosage of two pills two to three times daily at the onset of symptoms. Since it acts by inducing symptoms, anticipate a slight homeopathic aggravation (increase in symptoms). (See Introduction.)

For other remedies, see "Diarrhea," "Stomachache," "Flu."

ITCHING, ANAL (PRURITUS ANI)

THIS IS an unignorable itch around the anal area. The cause is often pinworms. A crack or redness at the anal opening caused by a sensitivity to a food ingested in the previous three days (milk, citrus, peaches, coffee) may also explain the symptoms. Candida is another possible cause of rectal itching. See "Pinworms," "Allergies," "Diaper Rash," "Candidiasis."

ITCHING (PRURITUS), RASH, POISON IVY, POISON OAK, HIVES

PRURITUS, OR itching, is the most common skin complaint. It can be caused by insect bites and stings, allergies, poison ivy or oak, sunburn, dry skin, or wet diapers. (See "Insect Bites and Stings," "Sunburn," "Diaper Rash.") Generalized itching over a large area of the body that lasts more than a week can also be a symptom of systemic disease requiring a doctor's attention. Possibilities includes diabetes mellitus, hypothyroidism, gout, leukemia, lymphoma (cancer of the lymph nodes), infection by parasites, kidney failure, and liver disease.

Rashes are skin eruptions that can vary from flat macules to bumpy warts and blisters. *Poison ivy* and *poison oak* are contact rashes that create a stinging, burning, itchy sensation wherever the irritating leaf touches the skin. Some children who love carrots and beta-carotene-containing foods will develop a yellow tint to the skin that may be confused with a rash. This condition is not serious, but if a child's skin and whites of the eyes turn yellow, a bile problem is indicated and a pediatric investigation is needed. (See "Jaundice.")

Hives are raised, whitish welts on the skin surrounded by a red rash. A common allergic reaction, they are usually quite itchy and may last from minutes to several days before going away.

Hives, along with other symptoms such as fever, nausea, abdominal cramps, and shortness of breath after a bee sting, insect bite, or drug injection, are indicative of anaphylaxis, a severe shock to the immune system requiring prompt medical attention.

 Drug Treatment

A SKIN rash typically represents the body's attempt to expel irritants. Histamine is released in this process. Over-the-counter anti-itch products may contain antihistamines, corticosteroids, local anesthetics, or counterirritants.

Corticosteroids are the most effective option for itch relief, but not the safest. Steroid creams (hydrocortisone and hydrocortisone acetate) work by inhibiting the body's elimination of irritants and preventing the release of histamine. If the irritant itself isn't removed, however, the rash is liable to come back in full force when the drug is stopped, an example of the "rebound effect" plaguing many drugs. Worse, when inflammation is reduced by suppressing the immune system, resistance to infection is lowered at the same time. The result can be secondary infection, including boils and thrush. If steroids are used to treat skin disorders caused by infection, much more severe infections may result, which can spread over large areas or produce ugly skin ulcers. Other potential adverse effects of topical steroids include allergic reactions, irreversible marks on the skin, unwanted hair growth, and acne. If used on children's skin, or in large amounts by adults, the drugs can enter the circulatory system and reach the pituitary, where they can have systemic effects like those seen with systemic steroids. **If the cream does not work after a week, or if the rash returns after the cream is stopped, consult a doctor.**[171] Best is to avoid cortisone creams on the skin.

Antihistamines taken in liquid or chewable tablet form immediately after a sting, bite, or exposure to poison ivy or poison oak can block the histamine receptors before they have time to release their itch-provoking hormone. Antihistamines applied to the skin can also relieve itching.

Other over-the-counter itch remedies are local anesthetics—drugs with active ingredients ending in "-caine." Their main drawback is that they can cause sensitivity reactions in susceptible people. Counter-irritants like camphor, menthol, and phenol seem to work by causing a mild irritation at other skin sites, diverting the pain receptors at the site of irritation. **Caution: Phenol can cause serious skin burns and, if swallowed, can cause internal injury, even in very weak concentrations. Keep it away from children and never use it to treat diaper rash.**[172]

 The Natural Approach: Treating the Cause

THERE ARE safe natural alternatives to drugs for soothing itching. One is the herb calendula. Weleda makes a high-quality line of children's products, including a calendula baby cream for irritated skin, diaper rash, and sores; a calendula baby lotion for diaper rash and skin rashes; and an all-natural, all-organic baby oil, baby soap, and burn-care ointment.

Clays may be applied to the skin as drawing salves to pull out toxins and relieve pain. Options include bentonite clay, kaolin clay, French green clay, and Aztec Secret by Aztec Corporation. Black Ointment by Nature's Way also pulls out splinters and slivers of glass.

For hives, try Hyland's homeopathic combination Hives.

For poison oak or poison ivy, good homeopathic combination products include Contact Allergies by Molecular Biologicals and Itch Nix by Quantum. The homeopathic remedy Rhus tox will quiet the rash in just a few hours. A tea of Calendula and Grindelia is also soothing. Undress the exposed child and bathe with soap and water as soon as possible after exposure. Wash the clothes thoroughly as well, as they can cause an outbreak in anyone who handles them.

An effective treatment for itching and excess dryness of the skin (a major cause of itching) is the wet dressing. Wet dressings work because the evaporating water cools and gently cleans the skin. To apply a wet dressing, soak a layer of gauze or thin cloth in water. (Diluted Burow's solution is sometimes recommended, but it contains high amounts of aluminum that may be absorbed by broken or inflamed skin.) Apply the wet gauze to the irritated area. Soak and reapply the cloth every two or three minutes for fifteen to thirty minutes. The procedure can be repeated several times a day. If itching covers an area too large for wet dressings, try a cool bath. Cool water constricts blood vessels. Avoid warm baths, which can increase vasodilation and itching.[173]

For dry skin, essential fatty acids (EFAs) can also help. Children with dry skin are likely to be getting insufficient EFAs in their diets. Child Life makes a product called Essential Fatty Acids in liquid form that is easy for kids to take. Good topical remedies for dry skin are evening primrose oil or shark-liver oil (500 milligrams or one to two capsules at bedtime for both).

Here are some nondrug suggestions for taking the itch out of mosquito bites:

1. Make a paste from unseasoned meat tenderizer and water. Apply to the bite and leave on for thirty minutes.

2. Coat the bite with fresh papaya, which contains an enzyme that neutralizes venom.

3. Rub the juice from the flowers and leaves of a honeysuckle vine into the bite.

4. Moisten the skin and sprinkle ordinary table salt on it.

5. Dab the skin with toothpaste.[174]

For natural ways to avoid bites, see "Insect Bites and Stings."

JAUNDICE

JAUNDICE IS characterized by a yellow tint to the skin and whites of the eyes, caused by high blood levels of bilirubin, a breakdown product of red blood cells. Before birth, most of the fetus's bilirubin passes through the placenta and is excreted by the mother's liver. After birth, the baby's liver must do this work unaided. Several days may pass before bilirubin can be eliminated faster than it is produced. During this time it can build up in the blood and cause jaundice. Premature babies are often jaundiced because their immature livers take longer to adjust to the work of elimination. While some degree of jaundice is normal and harmless, if bilirubin levels get too high, they can be toxic to the brain. High bilirubin levels may also indicate blood-group incompatibility between mother and child, infection, or other problems. See "Hepatitis."

The ingestion of many yellow fruits and vegetables, especially carrots, can give the skin a yellow carotene color that may be mistaken for jaundice. The difference is that the yellow color from fruits and vegetables shows only on the thick skin (the palms of the hands and soles of the feet), never in the whites of the eyes. If the whites of the eyes are yellow, look into liver abnormalities; a blood test for liver enzymes can distinguish between the two.

 Treatment

IN THE hospital, abnormally high bilirubin levels are treated with phototherapy (fluorescent light) to bring them within a safe range. The light alters bilirubin in the skin so that it can more easily be excreted by the infant. Eye patches are used to protect the baby's eyes. At home, expose the child to a few hours of indirect sunshine each day (through a glass window or outside in the shade) to help clear up jaundice.[175]

KNOCK-KNEES

THIS IS a common knee condition in children from about two to four and a half years of age. When knock-kneed children are in the standing position with the knees just touching, about two inches of space separate the ankle bones. Shoe salesmen will sometimes recommend special shoes with an inner sole lift to correct the situation, but the treatment is expensive and is not very effective. Fortunately, in 60 percent of children, the condition resolves without treatment by about six years of age just from normal growth. For those children with persistent, severe knock-knees, an orthopedist may prescribe braces.

LEAD POISONING (See Heavy-metal Poisoning)

LEFT-HANDEDNESS

AT ONE time, children who showed a tendency to be left-handed were disciplined to learn to use the right. This process not only proved frustrating but was later suspected to cause psychological damage to the child. Left-handedness is now linked with being right-brain dominant. People who are intuitive with form, balance, dimensions, and visual integrations tend to be right-brain-dominant.

A fairly reliable method of determining right- or left-handedness in infants is to compare the respective widths of the thumbnails (or the big toenails). If the right nail is broader, the child usually turns out to be right-handed; if the left nail is broader, left-handed.

> ### Stuttering Linked to
> ### Changing Dominant Hands
>
> The wife of author Dr. Smith was left-handed but had been encouraged at school to learn to write with her right hand. She found this experience quite stymying and began to stutter. When she returned to using her left hand, the stuttering stopped. As an adult, her artistic side manifested in a love of art and a successful career as an interior decorator.

LICE (See Head Lice)

LIVER DISEASE (See Hepatitis)

LYME DISEASE, TICK BITES

LYME DISEASE is a flulike bacterial infection induced by the bite of an infected black-legged tick. In cases that come to the practitioner without a diagnosis, the major problem is determining the cause of an elusive set of symptoms. The complaints of Lyme-disease victims tend to change from day to day. They can feel great one day and wretched the next. The illness is liable to be misdiagnosed or branded as psychological. The clearest early sign of the disease is a bull's-eye-shaped rash appearing within days or weeks of the tick bite; but this sign is often missed, and other symptoms imitate other diseases. In children as well as adults, every muscle, joint, organ, and tissue may have symptoms showing involvement. Early symptoms of Lyme disease can include muscle and joint aches and swelling, headache, stiff neck, overwhelming fatigue, fever, facial paralysis (Bell's palsy), meningitis, and (less commonly) visual disturbances and heart abnormalities. Late-stage symptoms include intermittent or chronic arthritis and neurological conditions such as confusion and memory loss.[176]

 Drug Treatment

STANDARD DRUG treatment consists of a three-week to month-long course of antibiotics in the initial stage, which must sometimes be repeated; in later stages, treatment is with an intravenous antibiotic, which can be quite disruptive and toxic to the body. Doctors caution that this course should be pursued only when the case is advanced and the diagnosis is definitive. In light of the difficult diagnosis, the patient runs the risk of being subjected to quite toxic drugs for the wrong underlying condition. New drug recommendations include oral antibiotics given at the time of exposure, to prevent the bacteria (called Borrelia) from dividing.

 Homeopathic Treatment

A LESS toxic alternative is homeopathic treatment, which can be used without a definitive diagnosis because the remedies have no dangerous side effects. If the remedy is not the correct one for the patient's condition, it will simply have no effect. Experimentation with these remedies can be used, in fact, to establish an otherwise tentative diagnosis. Homeopathic remedies are not only nontoxic but have proven effective in cases where antibiotics failed.

Hundreds of cases of Lyme disease have been referred by a medical office to Dr. Walker after the patients' symptoms returned following treatment with antibiotics. The drugs simply had not worked. They had suppressed rather than cured the disease, and had thrown off the natural balance of the body in the meantime. The remedy that resolved these patients' symptoms was a formulation of homeopathic Borrelia given as series therapy. The recommended protocol was a single dose in strengths varying from 200x to 5x taken every three days for a month.

For patients with recurring Lyme symptoms, who have had multiple courses of antibiotics, or who have been reinfected from new bites, higher potentcies should be used. Borrelia is available from Deseret in both 10m and 1m potencies. These are given from high potency to low potency (10m followed by 1m a week later), followed by the Deseret series box (200 to 5x). For a first-time exposure, caught before symptoms occur, the whole series is not necessary; Deseret Lyme drops can boost the immune system to stop the disease before it advances. Give ten drops three times daily.

 Preventive Measures

IF YOU cannot avoid tick-infested areas, minimize bite risk by protecting your child's arms and legs with long sleeves and long pants tucked into socks or boots, and use insect repellents. Permethrin-containing insect repellents can be applied to pants, socks, and shoes. The conventionally recommended DEET-containing repellents, however, are not ideal for exposed skin, since DEET is very toxic. Effective DEET-free herbal bug repellents are now on the market. A homeopathic remedy called Biting Insects by Molecular Biologicals is also quite effective. For other options, see "Insect Bites and Stings."

MALABSORPTION

THIS IS a condition of the intestinal tract that selectively inhibits the absorption of some nutrients essential to health. Food sensitivities may so damage the intestinal lining that it cannot absorb even the nutrients from healthy foods. Milk, soy, corn, wheat, eggs, peanuts, and seafood are the main food triggers; but the condition's underlying cause may be treatment with antibiotics. The drugs destroy beneficial bacteria necessary for digestion along with harmful bacteria, allowing the yeast *Candida albicans* to grow and preventing proper absorption of nutrients. To avoid this result, always give acidophilus bifidus cultures following any antibiotic used for more than a few days. Child Life makes a "Friendly Flora/Bifidus" for kids. Nutrition Now makes a chewable raspberry-flavored acidophilus tablet that contains no dairy or whey, along with a powdered acidophilus product for children.

MALOCCLUSION OF THE TEETH
(See Dental Problems)

MEASLES

MEASLES ACTUALLY comes in five forms, all due to viruses.

The form commonly referred to as *measles* lasts a week, produces a hard cough, and can lead to complications. For this reason, a vaccine has been developed to prevent it. However, contracting the disease gives permanent immunity, while the measles vaccine does not;[177] and immunizations may contribute to the development of autoimmune diseases. For discussion, see "Immunizations."

German measles or *rubella* (three-day measles) does not lead to complications, except when a woman contracts it in the first three months of pregnancy, in which case it can cause deafness in her baby.

Roseola usually occurs at about one year of age. It can include a rather alarming fever (104 to 106 degrees) for seventy-two hours, sometimes with febrile convulsions. When the fever drops, a flat red rash appears (mainly on the trunk) and lasts for three more days. Alarmed parents usually want treatment, but an emergency white blood count will reassure them that they are dealing only with a virus and that home care to make the child comfortable is all that is required.

Duke's disease is a rare form of measles characterized by fever and a rash.

Another rare form is *fifth disease,* involving a faint rash on the arms without fever. It lasts about four days and is unproblematic but can be confused with allergy.

 Natural Alternatives

IF TAKEN at the onset of symptoms, high doses of vitamin C and echinacea can help the immune system fight infection. (For provisos, see "Colds.") Other herbal options include olive-leaf extract and elderberry, both of which are natural antivirals and antibacterials. Elderberry comes in chewable flavors for children.

Viracin by CompliMed is a combination homeopathic remedy useful for speeding recovery from measles. Homeopathic remedies for specific symptom patterns include:

> Belladonna: if the child is hot and restless with a high fever
> Arsenicum alba: if the child is debilitated, restless, and experiences an aggravation of symptoms around midnight
> Euphrasia: for inflammation of the eyes, nose, and mucous membranes, with sneezing
> Bryonia: to cut short the disease at first onset

MENINGITIS

MENINGITIS IS an inflammation of the meninges, the membrane that covers the brain and spinal cord. It requires immediate medical attention. Bacterial forms of the disease are life-threatening if not treated, although viral forms are comparatively mild. Onset can be sudden or gradual. Early diagnosis is important. Symptoms include a severe headache, and stiffness and pain in the neck or back; a high fever, severe vomiting, and convulsions may also occur. The white blood count is elevated and there are white blood cells in the spinal fluid.

Conventional Treatment

PEDIATRICIANS TREAT meningitis immediately and vigorously with an antibiotic specific to the bacteria.

Natural Support Therapies

HOMEOPATHIC REMEDIES that can help relieve symptoms include Apis 200 (for acute infection), Belladonna 200 (for a very high temperature with severe headache), and Cuprum metallicum (for nausea and vomiting). The German company Staufen also makes excellent homeopathic remedies. Comparable series therapy is available in the United States from Deseret.

Olive-leaf extract is a powerful herbal antibacterial and antiviral that can speed healing. Elderberry is another option.

MENSTRUAL PROBLEMS, CRAMPS, PUBERTY IN GIRLS

GIRLS TODAY are beginning menstruation earlier than their mothers did. Normal ages range anywhere from eight to sixteen. Some authorities attribute earlier onset to the growth hormones fed to cows and chickens, which wind up in the milk, meat, and eggs that children ingest. Other authorities point to the estrogenic effects of pesticides and chemicals in food. Whatever the cause, mothers now need to begin those mother/daughter talks earlier. Don't wait until your daughter is thirteen or fourteen—you may need to begin at seven or eight. You want her to hear the facts from you before she gets the distorted version from her friends. These talks also represent an opportunity for an open dialogue that can mature into a lifelong bond.

Explain to your daughter that her breasts will start to develop and pubic hair will appear; that there may be twinges in the abdomen and a little egg-white-like discharge during ovulation; that irritability and mood swings are normal with menstruation. Let her know that hormonal development varies. Some girls start their periods early, others late. Explain that breast buds are not tumors but are budding breasts, and that one breast may be larger than the other (this is common). Buy sanitary pads for her so she'll feel prepared. Tampons hold toxins inside the body, increasing the risk of toxic shock syndrome, and are therefore not recommended except when swimming or when pads are otherwise inappropriate. Pads should be unbleached. Bleached pads contain toxic dioxins that have been linked to endometriosis.

For remedies for mood swings, see "Premenstrual Syndrome (PMS)."

 ## Conventional Treatment for Menstrual Cramps

FOR MENSTRUAL cramps, the conventional approach is painkillers like Midol and Advil. But these drugs merely mask the symptom without addressing the real problem, and women often find they need more and more to get the same results. The drugs work by inhibiting a natural function, the synthesis of prostaglandins in the body. The body compensates by making more prostaglandins the next month, and more the next.

Natural Alternatives

PERMANENT CURE has been reported from the use of homeopathic remedies for menstrual cramps, which correct the underlying imbalance in the body's energetic field. Cyclease by Boiron is particularly good. Relief is usually obtained with the first period, and after a few period cycles, all cramps disappear. Women report that this remedy has changed their lives, and the product is quite safe even for young girls. Dosage is one to three times daily starting the day before the period is expected. The remedy may be taken up to every hour during cramping.

Mag phos, a cell salt, is another effective alternative, taken from the day before until the second day of the menstrual period.

Contessa by MPI is a homeopathic female tonic that will regulate the period and eliminate cramps when taken over several months.

If these remedies don't work, consult a homeopath for an appropriate constitutional remedy.

Effective Chinese herbal remedies are also available. Chinese doctors note that menstrual cramps vary in degree and type. They say that when the blood is dark with clots, last month's blood has stayed in the tubes. The more stagnation there is in the body and the darker and more clotted the blood, the worse the cramps. Relief requires "moving the blood." The Chinese patent formula to achieve this result is Hsiao Yao Wan. The dose is eight pills three times daily from ovulation to menstruation.

For swelling of the breasts before the menstrual period, the homeopathic remedy is Sepia 30c.

When young girls' breasts produce milk, use Pulsatilla 30c.

For anemia resulting from long, heavy periods, use Ferrum phos taken as a cell salt in a 6x potency three to four times daily. It will build the blood over a period of several months.

MIGRAINE HEADACHE (See Headaches)

MONONUCLEOSIS, EPSTEIN-BARR VIRUS

INFECTIOUS MONONUCLEOSIS has been attributed to the Epstein-Barr virus, but the whole syndrome remains a mystery. Formerly called "the kissing disease," "mono" frequently occurs in adolescents and young adults living together; yet researchers have been unable to successfully transmit it from one volunteer to another. Symptoms come on gradually, with fever, sore throat, general discomfort, loss of appetite, and headache that can be severe. The lymph glands gradually swell, and the spleen and liver are frequently enlarged. The disease can last from one to eight weeks, after which the patient may feel abnormally weak and tired for weeks or months. Symptoms may then recur or may develop into chronic fatigue syndrome, a condition that can persist for years. At least one hundred thousand cases of mononucleosis occur in the United States each year.[178]

 Conventional Treatment

THE CONSERVATIVE recommendation is simply to wait mono out, with bed rest, a soft diet, fluids, and aspirin. Antibiotics don't affect the course of the disease, but they often are prescribed before a definite diagnosis. The result can be repeated courses of different and stronger antibiotics, with a corresponding weakening of the body's immune defenses. Aggressive doctors are now also giving steroids for mono, suppressing the immune system even further and preventing the body from healing. Many adult patients with chronic fatigue syndrome report a history of mono followed by antibiotics, compounded by some stressor (such as an injury or personal crisis).

Alternative Treatment

A HOMEOPATHIC remedy called Mononucleosis, made by the German company, Staufen, can knock out the condition early and permanently. Comparable series therapy is available in the United States from Deseret. Because the disease has a tendency to evolve into chronic fatigue syndrome, the remedy is recommended even for people who had mono years earlier. Those who take it are often amazed at how much better they feel afterward, even when they thought they were well.

A gemmotherapy called Tamarisk by Dolisos is an herbal remedy good for relieving the symptoms of mononucleosis and other conditions in which the child is weak and run-down.

High-dose vitamin C given daily can also help speed recovery. The dose can be increased until sloppy bowel movements result (5 to 10 grams daily).

Natural Remedies Prevent Lost School Days

A nineteen-year-old college student was quite sick with mononucleosis. He was falling asleep in class and had been told to stay out of the classroom because he was so ill, but that meant he would lose an entire semester of classwork. The young man was treated with the Staufen mononucleosis remedy. To his amazement, all his symptoms were gone in two days, allowing him to finish the college semester.

A second case involved a fourteen-year-old girl who was still tired, pale, and missing school four months after contracting mono. After two weeks' treatment with Mononucleosis by Staufen, she experienced a remarkable recovery and returned to school quite healthy.

MORNING SICKNESS (See Nausea)

MOTION SICKNESS (See Nausea)

MUMPS

MUMPS IS a viral infection in the salivary glands that causes the parotid gland to swell and push up the earlobe. Swelling may also show under the chin, or under the area of the molars. The infection sometimes proceeds to the pancreas and causes abdominal pain and nausea. Rarely, it may go to the brain and produce an excruciating headache, fever, and general feeling of misery. In adults, mumps may also go to the testes or ovaries. A mumps vaccine is available that gives immunity, but duration is not known. Allowing the disease to run its course will develop a permanent immunity.

 Natural Remedies

VITAMIN C in large doses will help the child with mumps to remain comfortable while his immune system is learning to resist the infection.

Homeopathy also helps. Viracin by CompliMed is a combination remedy that speeds recovery. For mumps in the acute phase, alternate Mercuris iodum with Belladonna every half hour till the acute phase is over. Then continue Belladonna four times daily until the patient is well. For mumps with severe ear pain, give the homeopathic remedy Pulsatilla.

MUSCLE CRAMPS AND SPASMS, CHARLEY HORSE, GROWING PAINS

MUSCLE PAINS and cramps can have a variety of causes, including:

1. Low serum potassium: from vomiting or diarrhea, or because the child is eating insufficient fresh foods

2. Low serum calcium: from insufficient calcium intake from milk or other calcium sources

3. Insufficient oxygenation to the cells: from high altitudes, long-distance running, or in asthmatic children

4. Lactic acid buildup: from overexercising

A *charley horse* is a cramp in the leg muscles (usually the calf), typically occurring at night. In children, it generally follows a day of physical exercise and is caused by an accumulation of lactic acid, a by-product of muscular activity.

Growing pains typically strike in the evening and result because the child's bones are literally stretching and growing.

 Natural Remedies

THE HOMEOPATHIC remedy for relieving leg spasms is Cuprum metallicum. Effective combination homeopathics are also available: Dolisos makes one called Leg Cramps, as does Hyland's. Sportenine by Boiron stops lactic acid buildup and reduces recovery time from muscle cramps from heavy exercise.

To relieve muscle cramps from low potassium levels, the solution is more potassium. An effervescent vitamin C called Emer'gen-C containing 800 milligrams of potassium is good, and kids love its fizziness and multiple flavors.

For muscle cramps due to insufficient calcium, increase the child's calcium intake, either in foods or from supplements. Nutrition Now makes a chewable calcium for kids. An advantage of Calc carb, the homeopathic alternative, is that unlike many calcium supplements, it will not cause constipation.

Take calcium or potassium supplements before bed to help relieve muscle spasms occurring at night.

A remedy that works over the space of about a half hour to relieve charley horses in the calves is to take 500 milligrams of magnesium at the onset of the cramp. Liquid supplements work faster than tablets.

If magnesium and calcium supplements are not soluble enough to help the muscles relax, acidify the system to increase their solubility. Many pregnant women will send their husbands out in the middle of the night for ice cream, adding as an afterthought, "Don't forget the pickles!" Pregnant women seem to know instinctively that acidifying the calcium makes it more absorbable for them and the fetus. The sense of taste can be an accurate barometer of the body's needs. If a teaspoon of apple cider vinegar in an eight-ounce glass of water tastes good and sweet, the body probably needs it. The system has become too alkaline due to an excess of sodium in the system. Ammonium chloride is another acidifier, though not all druggists carry it.

For muscle pain from low oxygenation, Cellular Oxygenator by PHP is good. This remedy also works for altitude sickness, particularly if taken just before going to higher altitudes.

For breathing problems, shortness of breath, or asthma from over-exercising, black-currant-seed oil can open the lungs and increase breathing capacity. Many athletes take two capsules before a run or match to make breathing easier.

To relieve growing pains, try homeopathic Calc carb 30c.

Muscle Cramps Relieved with Natural Remedy

Eleven-year-old Tommy loved baseball, but he wound up in tears at night from the muscle cramps he got in his legs after playing baseball all day. Leg Cramps by Hyland's, a homeopathic remedy (two taken in the evening), allowed him to sleep through the night without leg cramping.

NAIL BITING, THUMB SUCKING, PACIFIERS

THESE "NERVOUS" habits have been attributed to a variety of causes, including stresses in the home or school, or just from growing up; insufficient sucking at the breast or bottle in infancy; and an attempt to ignore intestinal disturbances by rhythmically sucking and biting. Parents' efforts to stop the child may merely reinforce the habit by allowing it to become a source of special attention; but some effort should be made to control persistent thumb sucking, since the habit can push the front teeth forward into a bucktoothed position. Children who bite and suck are also more likely to swallow pinworm eggs transferred from their peers, thus inducing another stressor in the body.

Nail biting can indicate pinworms. Children treated for pinworms have been observed to stop biting their nails.

 Natural Alternatives

FOR YOUNG children, pacifiers can help discourage the use of thumb or fingers as a sucking device and relaxer. Pacifiers are nipple-shaped devices, usually made of rubber or plastic, used to satisfy an infant's sucking needs. The bony appendages of the fingers tend to push the teeth around more forcefully than rubber or plastic. Pacifiers are typically continued for the first year or two, after which the need for them falls off, but there is no harm in their prolonged use. The child will usually abandon the pacifier when in nursery school or kindergarten due to peer pressure. Interestingly, breast-fed babies rarely need pacifiers.

For a young girl with a thumb addiction, try painting the nails with bright fingernail polish. Vanity may keep her from biting her pretty nails.

NASOLACRIMAL DUCT OBSTRUCTION

IN THIS condition, one or both eyes of the newborn are full of green or yellow pus because the tears cannot flow from the surface of the eyes into the duct that carries them into the nasal cavity. The condition is easily diagnosed.

Conventional Treatment

AN ANTIBIOTIC ointment may be used to control the condition. (For downsides of antibiotics, see "Immunity.") If the condition persists, an ophthalmologist may have to pass a probe through the duct to open it. Some obstructions are due to fibrous or bony growths.

Natural Alternatives

OFTEN THESE obstructions will clear of their own accord if the duct is massaged so that pressure on the skin at the inner corner of the eye opens the duct. Optique Eyedrops by Boiron, containing homeopathic Calendula, may also help.

NAUSEA, VOMITING, MOTION SICKNESS, MORNING SICKNESS

NAUSEA AND vomiting usually represent the body's attempt to get rid of harmful bacteria or other toxins. In those cases, do not suppress vomiting. Other causes of nausea and vomiting include motion sickness, stress, pregnancy (morning sickness), migraine headache, and allergies. Nausea and vomiting may also be caused by drugs, including antibiotics, narcotic painkillers like codeine, birth-control pills, and prescription asthma medications. Iron supplements and salt substitutes have been implicated as well.

Projectile vomiting is the forceful emptying of the stomach associated with intestinal obstruction. Its occurrence in an infant under one month old is a clue that the child has pyloric stenosis, an obstruction due to swollen muscles at the outlet of the stomach, causing its contents to shoot a few feet out. Surgery is usually required in those cases.

Nausea can indicate a serious condition, including ulcers, colorectal cancer, diabetes, Crohn's disease, meningitis, and mononucleosis, among other suspects. If your child is vomiting blood or has abdominal pain, headache, dizziness, fever, or a racing heartbeat, or if the vomiting lasts more than four hours, consult your pediatrician.

For nausea from chemical poisoning, see "Poisoning."

 Drug Treatment

THE FDA has declared that no over-the-counter drugs are safe and effective for treating nausea and vomiting. There are drugs that work, but they either require a prescription or the FDA restricts their over-the-counter sale to treating motion sickness. Motion sickness isn't caused by something the body is trying to get rid of, so suppressing it with drugs doesn't involve retaining potential poisons. Drowsiness is a side effect of these drugs.

 ## Natural Remedies

FOR MOTION sickness or car sickness, a particularly good homeopathic remedy is Travel Sickness by Dolisos (two pills three to four times daily).

The Sea-Band, an elastic band placed on the wrist, is another safe, effective, and easy motion-sickness alternative. It puts pressure on one of the major acupuncture points of the body. It is particularly good for restless children who complain about getting sick in the car.

Ginger and a Chinese formula called Bao Ji Wan are other effective motion-sickness remedies. Ginger helps relieve nausea in general. It can either be taken as capsules or drunk as a tea.

Pill Curing is an excellent Chinese herbal remedy for settling the stomach after a large meal or when the food feels stuck in the mid-section. This remedy can also quell motion sickness without inducing drowsiness.

Effective homeopathic remedies are also available for nausea and vomiting caused by indigestion. One is Carbo Veg 6c. The dosage is three tablets every fifteen minutes. For severe upset, up to six doses may be given.

For cramps, nausea, vomiting, and pain caused by food poisoning, Arsenicum alba 6x is recommended (two pills every fifteen minutes, up to six doses). Another option is Salmonella 200x. Often a single dose will relieve severe cramping and nausea.

For morning sickness, homeopathics are the only remedies that can be recommended during pregnancy with absolute confidence in their safety. Homeopathic remedies work on a vibrational rather than a chemical level.

(See Introduction.) A great homeopathic remedy for morning sickness is Symphoricarpus. Another option is a homeopathic combination by Molecular Biologicals called Nausea. Herbs should not be used during pregnancy, with the exception of red raspberry leaf, which can be sipped as a tea during morning sickness and is good for use during the last six weeks of pregnancy to strengthen and tone the uterus and prepare it for giving birth.

Contrary to popular belief, liquids—especially carbonated drinks—are hard for an upset stomach to keep down. A cracker or other dry food is better. You can drink colas or ginger ales, but they should be flat, at room temperature, and taken in small sips. Other good fluids are apple and grape juices drunk at room temperature. Citrus juices are not as good, since their acidity can irritate the stomach and they often contain solid pulp that is hard to digest.[179]

The homeopathic remedy for projectile vomiting is Ipecac.

Projectile Vomiting Cured with Homeopathic Remedy

A six-year-old boy had contracted a fever and had been projectile vomiting for a full day, shooting what appeared to be a huge quantity for such a small child halfway across the room. Homeopathic Ipecac stopped the vomiting immediately and dramatically.

NAVEL

THE NAVEL, or belly button, is either an "innie" or an "outie": Some are indentations and some protrude outward from the abdomen. This characteristic has nothing to do with the way the umbilical cord was tied at the time of delivery. Rather, in some newborns an inch or two of skin remains covering the cord, so when the cord remnant dries up and is absorbed, some extra skin protrudes. If the navel pooches out somewhat when the baby cries, a hernia is indicated. These protrusions will disappear in time and rarely need surgery, but some surgeons like to repair them before they disappear. (See "Hernia.")

NIGHT TERRORS, NIGHTMARES

THE CHILD who awakens suddenly in great fear, screaming, sobbing, mumbling, or having nightmares, is said to be suffering from night terrors. Nightmares and night terrors may have a variety of causes, including psychological stressors, a vivid imagination, and frightening movies or television shows. Children accept as real what their parents know to be "just a movie." One of the authors' children had night terrors for weeks after seeing the original *Ghostbusters* at the age of three, a movie her parents considered a comedy.

Nightmares can also be caused by low blood sugar. You might recognize this common scenario: Your child awakens in the middle of the night with a piercing scream, as if she has been attacked by an enormous bear. You rush to her bedroom and try to awaken and calm her. You notice she has broken out in a sweat, and when her eyes open, the pupils are dilated. Why? The fright is triggered by an adrenaline rush. Think back to what you fed her before bed. If it was milk and cookies or a bowl of ice cream (20 percent sugar), her blood sugar would rise and she would fall asleep. But her body would then react to the onslaught by producing insulin to push the sugar into the muscles and liver, and her blood sugar would fall. The reaction of the body to this apparent crisis is a release of adrenaline, with the same physical symptoms as if the body were under attack from some external threat. Adrenaline prepares the body for fight or flight. Nightmares can result.

Natural Remedies for Night Terrors

THE REMEDY for nightmares from low blood sugar is to provide a protein snack (chicken, fish, soy) at bedtime so the blood sugar rises and falls gradually over several hours. If the blood sugar does not fall too fast, adrenaline is not released. If low blood sugar is the source of the problem, the therapy should work the first night it is tried. See "Hypoglycemia."

A good Bach flower remedy for nightmares is Cherry Plum.

Effective homeopathic remedies include:

Aconitum: for nightmares or night terrors or fitful mumbling in the sleep

Spongia: for the child who wakes up in a fright, feeling suffocated

Belladonna: for the child who screams out in sleep

Chinese doctors attribute nightmares and night terrors to anemia. Blood deficiencies to the heart can give the child an unsettled feeling and cause nightmares. The remedy is to nourish the blood and heart. Ferrum phos is the homeopathic remedy to build the blood. For a Chinese herbal remedy, see an herbalist.

For aids to induce sleep, see "Insomnia."

NOSEBLEEDS

NOSEBLEEDS ARE common in children during cold, dry weather, during the hot summer, or after slight trauma. They are sometimes hard to stop. Nosebleeds that occur without trauma may be from dryness in the nose or from allergies. Milk sensitivity is a possible cause.

Home Remedies

Have the child sit down and lean slightly forward to prevent blood from running into the throat. Place cold, wet cloths on the nose to constrict the blood vessels. If blood is coming from only one nostril, press firmly at the top of that nostril. If both nostrils are bleeding, pinch the nostrils together for at least ten minutes; if bleeding continues, apply another ten minutes of pressure. If the bleeding is the result of direct injury to the nose, apply only gentle pressure.

Another alternative is to put a pledget of wet cotton or tissue into the bleeding nostril. Apply pressure from the outside, holding for ten minutes. Leave the pledget for another ten minutes, then slowly pull it out. Apply a greasy ointment to prevent another nosebleed from dried blood. Calendula and Hypericum ointment is good.

The homeopathic remedy for nosebleeds is the cell salt Ferrum phos 6x or 30c, three pills three times daily. Bioflavonoids and vitamin C orally may help increase capillary integrity.

If heavy bleeding persists, or if nosebleeds recur frequently, consult a physician. If frequent nosebleeds are due to allergies, you may need to track down and address the triggers. (See "Allergies.")

NUTRITION, NUTRITIONAL SUPPLEMENTS, INFANT FEEDING, MILK SUBSTITUTES

Children are finicky eaters. They are likely to disdain vegetables and lack the discipline to reject sugary and other junk foods. The average American child eats twice the recommended allotment of sugar every day, and one and a half times the recommended allotment of fat. As a result, childhood obesity is on the rise; and these intakes of empty calories are at the expense of the fruits, vegetables, and whole grains that should provide the nutrients necessary for proper growth and development. If children are eating junk food, they are not only burdened with a high toxic load but are getting insufficient vitamins, minerals, amino acids, and other nutrients. Health problems are being traced increasingly to nutritional deficiencies that can be corrected only by supplying these missing nutrients.

At one time, everything the body needed was furnished by the foods of the earth; but today, the earth seems to be as depleted as our bodies. Canning, irradiation, and other methods of preserving shelf life have decreased the biological value of our food. A report presented to the U.S. Department of Agriculture in 1936 concluded that our soils and their crops are so mineral-deficient that the only way to prevent and cure the resulting deficiency diseases is by taking mineral supplements, and that was more than half a century ago.[180] The situation has declined significantly since.

 ## Recommended Nutritional Supplementation

FOR BREAST-FED babies, few nutritional supplements are necessary; but some authorities feel the baby does not get enough vitamin D from breast milk. Just exposing the baby to the blue sky for ten to twenty minutes is considered sufficient to satisfy the vitamin-D requirement in the summer, but supplementation with 400 IU of the vitamin during the winter may be continued for a few years. While all the other essentials are usually in breast milk, the pediatrician may also recommend some B-vitamin drops to be safe. Much depends on the mother's health and her nutrient intake.

If the baby is being bottle-fed, check the formula for sufficient vitamins, minerals, and essential fatty acids. If it doesn't provide adequate vitamins and minerals, you should supplement daily. Ask your pediatrician for recommended brands of formula and vitamin and mineral drops.

For children past babyhood, a good daily multiple vitamin and mineral supplement is recommended. Not all brands are equally good. Natural is better than synthetic, and nutrients need to be in proper balance and in an absorbable form. Particularly good brands include

Nutrition Now, NF Formulas, and Child Life. For the younger child, supplementation comes in chewable tablets; for the older child, it comes as tablets or capsules to be swallowed whole. Specific supplements are also recommended in this book for specific disease conditions.

 Introduction of Solid Food

BREAST MILK is the best food for human babies. (See "Breast-feeding.") The fact that teeth do not erupt until about eight to ten months of age suggests that Mother Nature did not intend babies to have solid food until that time. In their zeal to start solid foods, pediatricians have caused babies to acquire sensitivities to foods introduced when the gut was immature. The more common allergenic foods—eggs, citrus, tomatoes, nut butters, even soy products—should be left for introduction until after the first birthday.

At one time, medical school teaching was that pediatricians should instruct mothers to introduce some rice cereal into their babies' diets at one month old. The theory was that this would help the baby sleep through the night, but it was not borne out in practice. Babies sleep through the night when they stop growing so fast that the amount of milk they can swallow during the day is insufficient to prevent hunger at night. If the baby can be fed every two or three hours during the day, he will sometimes sleep six hours at night.

Probably the safest food to introduce at ten months of age is steamed zucchini, one of the least allergenic foods. Applesauce, steamed carrots, and puréed vegetables can follow. The grains—wheat, corn, rice, oats—are best left out of the diet until one year of age or later. A prudent guideline is to introduce a new food no more frequently that once a week. Avoid sweet sugary foods—desserts, cake, ice cream (which is 20 percent sugar)—until a special birthday. Sweet foods are addictive and cause dental caries, since the minerals necessary to prevent tooth decay are deficient in them.

Avoiding Junk Food

IT IS up to parents to regulate children's diets. The sugar habit is an addiction: the more you give it, the more kids crave it. If you don't want your children to live on junk food, don't keep it in the house and don't give them free rein to buy it. One of the authors was asked for help with a boy who had ADD (attention deficit disorder). His mother said he typically ate a whole loaf of white bread for dinner—nothing else. She allowed it because "it's all he will eat." Compare this case to a woman who was raised as a Seventh Day Adventist and is now, at fifty, the picture of health. "My parents let us eat whatever we wanted, whenever we wanted," she said. "They told us to go out in the garden and eat whatever we wanted."

Keep the house stocked with fresh fruits and vegetables and learn tasty ways to serve them. Give children's foods creative names like "ants on a log" (fresh celery painted with peanut butter and lined with raisins); call your banana smoothies "banana milk shakes." Children raised on healthy food won't crave junk food and will find it less appealing than the nutrient-rich foods of their youth.

 ## Drinks and Sugar Substitutes

HONEY IS a healthy substitute for sugar, but infants under a year old should not be fed products containing honey due to the remote risk of acquiring botulism. Their digestive enzymes are not strong enough to detoxify the botulism spores.[181] Honey left in the teeth can also cause tooth decay.

Fruit juice can be overdone as well. A 1999 study found that fruit juice can cause restlessness, gas, and stomach distress in infants, who have difficulty breaking down carbohydrates; yet 90 percent of babies drink some type of fruit juice by one year of age. The sugars in fruit juice also contribute to major distortions of insulin balance that lead to hormone and neurotransmitter shifts, increasing a child's risk of ear infections, ADHD (attention deficit hyperactivity disorder),[182] and allergies. Gatorade can't be recommended, since it is high in sodium and contains artificial food coloring along with sugar.

Aspartame (Nutrasweet) should also be avoided. See "Aspartame (Artificial Sweetener) Addiction." The best thirst quencher for adults and children remains pure water. F. Batmanghelidj, M.D., in *Your Body's Many Cries for Water,* points to a modern epidemic of diseases that he attributes to dehydration, resulting from the mistaken assumption that our need for water has been satisfied by satisfying our thirst with other beverages. He says we need half our body's weight in ounces of water per day—not soft drinks, juices, coffee, or tea, but plain (filtered or bottled) water. Thus a child weighing sixty-four pounds would need thirty-two ounces, or four glasses, daily. Wait half an hour before meals and two and a half hours after meals for these heavy water doses, to avoid diluting the digestive juices.[183]

 ## Food Substitutes for Children Sensitive to Milk and Wheat

FOR CHILDREN with allergies, asthma, or frequent colds or flus, dairy products can worsen them by thickening mucus secretions. However, if you eliminate dairy products from the diet, you need to find alternative sources of calcium. Milk is considered the ideal calcium source in the United States, but it is actually an insignificant part of the diet for most indigenous populations, whose rates of osteoporosis (bone loss) are substantially lower than in industrialized populations. Readily available fresh milk is a product of technological civilization and of refrigeration. For many people in underdeveloped countries, calcium is provided by vegetables (including roots, tubers, seeds, and the greens of root vegetables) and by soy milk and its solid counterpart, tofu.

The least allergenic milk substitute is rice milk, as in Rice Dream. Rice Dream ice-cream bars are a treat children enjoy. Soy milk is another possible milk substitute, but it should be used only in small amounts, since too much soy taken on a daily basis could inhibit the lymph glands from draining well. Limit intake of soy products to one a day. Soy yogurt and soy ice-cream bars are favorites of children, but they shouldn't be served along with soy milk, soy hot dogs, and tofu in the same day.

Calcium can be obtained from nutritional supplements. Chewable calcium tablets are available (made by Nutrition Now).

Good substitutes for children who need to limit or avoid wheat products are also available. Ener'G makes a line of rice-flour products, including cookies and boxed ingredients that can be used for home baking. Good frozen wheat-free waffles are also available. Explore other options at your health food store.

OBSESSIVE-COMPULSIVE DISORDER
(See Depression)

OTITIS MEDIA (See Ear Infections)

OBESITY, OVERWEIGHT

OBESITY IS on the increase among children as well as adults. Defined as weight that is more than 30 percent above the ideal for one's height and age, obesity is estimated to affect 25 to 30 percent of American children before puberty and 18 to 25 percent of adolescents. It is a risk factor for chronic disease and associated mortality, and childhood is a critical period for its initiation.[184] A Canadian study found that the number of kids who qualified as obese went from about one in seven to almost one in four from 1981 to 1988, a time when significant changes occurred in children's lifestyles, including the invention of the TV remote, the proliferation of video games and computers, fewer kids walking to school, and the explosion of junk foods.[185]

A major risk factor for obesity in children is parental obesity. A child has an 80 percent chance of being obese when both parents are, and a 40 percent chance when only one parent is. When neither parent is obese, chances of childhood obesity are reduced to 7 percent. The association may not be due to heredity—bad family eating habits could also explain the link. Family factors contributing to the risk of childhood obesity include the mother's chosen method of feeding (such as short duration of breast-feeding) and early introduction of solid foods. Cultural habits also affect obesity in children, including pride in a fat baby, the belief that rapid weight gain in infancy demonstrates good health, reinforced overeating, prolonged and excessive amounts of bottle-feeding, lack of parental knowledge about food and feeding practices, and using food for reward, punishment, or comfort. Parents need not be concerned if their baby appears a little chunky, which is normal for children up to two years of age; but if the trend continues, some attention should be paid to the child's diet.

 Pharmaceutical Solutions

THE MEDICAL trend is to view obesity as a disease that should be treated with drugs. Prescription weight-loss drugs are now being tested even in children and teenagers.[186] One of these drugs, Xenical, works by reducing the absorption of dietary fat. A side effect is that it also limits intake of some vitamins, which can be a potentially serious problem in growing children. It can also cause excessive gas and urgent bowel movements. Another drug, Meridian, works by affecting chemicals in the brain involved in regulating appetite. Side effects include dry mouth, headache, insomnia, and constipation. The drugs are recommended only for acutely overweight kids.[187]

Over-the-counter diet aids are available for the mildly overweight. These drugs typically contain combinations of phenylpropanolamine (PPA), ephedrine derivatives, and caffeine, ingredients that are weaker than amphetamines but have similar chemical structures and reactions in the body. They stimulate the sympathethic nervous system, the "fight or flight" emergency system; and in high doses, they can produce psychotic-like side effects and hypertensive crises like amphetamines.[188]

 ### Natural Uppers: Ephedra/Ma Huang

THOUGH LESS hazardous than the pharmaceutical variety, some herbal diet pills also carry risks. The natural stimulant ephedrine (under the names *ma huang,* ephedra, or epitonin) has replaced amphetamines not only in "natural" diet aids but in herbal combinations popular among young people advertised as producing a "natural high." Over-dosing on natural ephedra, like on synthetic ephedrine, has been linked to heart attack, stroke, and sudden death, leading the FDA to consider banning or limiting the use of all ephedrine products both as weight loss and as bodybuilding aids. New York and Florida banned their sale after a twenty-year-old college student died following an overdose of an ephedrine-containing herbal product called Ultimate Xphoria.[189] However, a government report released in August 1999 said the FDA did not have the evidence it needed to impose restrictions.[190] Opponents counter that herbal ephedra is safer than the synthetic ephedrine and amphetamine products it has replaced both as diet aids and as recreational drugs.

Dietary Solutions

THE BEST solution remains dietary regulation. Dieting fads are as popular as ever, but many popular diets are of dubious merit. A low-calorie, low-fat diet is the most common diet plan. Ideally, it consists of cutting out junk foods and concentrating on fruits, vegetables, whole grains, and lean meats. Problems arise when dieters try to trick their taste buds with artificial sweeteners and fake fats (Olestra).

The Calorie Control Council reports that four out of five Americans now consume low-cal, sugar-free, or reduced-fat food and beverages containing these altered substances; yet Americans have gotten heavier, not lighter, since artificial sweeteners became popular. New evidence suggests that artificial sweeteners actually *cause* weight gain, by upsetting the body's natural insulin-regulating mechanisms. (See "Aspartame [Artificial Sweetener] Addiction.") Fat-free fat poses similar problems. Olestra was conditionally approved by the FDA for marketing in early 1996. Virtually identical to mineral oil, it is a laxative that depletes the body of fat-soluble vitamins and other essential nutrients if used habitually; and it can cause diarrhea and cramping, among other side effects. Fake fat is not calculated to work any better than fake sugar for producing weight loss. Low-fat foods often contain more calories than high-fat foods. The fat is simply replaced with sugar.[191] Moreover, some fat is needed in the diet. Hormones including estrogen, progesterone, testosterone, and the stress hormone cortisol are all made from cholesterol.

The safer course is to simply feed your child a balanced diet of natural foods in modest portions, reducing sugary and other junk foods. Overweight children and teens may crave food and eat large amounts of it because their bodies are seeking the minerals and vitamins not found in processed foods. The solution is to return to natural, whole, unprocessed foods without additives. Fake fats and sugars can fool the taste buds, but the body knows it needs real, wholesome fats and carbohydrates and will continue to crave them. To be well nourished, it needs essential fatty acids, complex carbohydrates, fiber, and a wide range of vitamins and minerals.

Digestive enzymes taken with meals can also help. Enzymes are necessary for proper nutrient absorption. Better yet is to get enzymes from their natural sources—especially raw fruits and vegetables—since they're lost in cooking, microwaving, and processing of foods.

Other factors in weight loss are the size and frequency of meals. Eating small amounts of food every two to three hours rather than three large meals a day helps keep some people from gaining. It prevents the blood sugar from falling too low, which would prompt the eating of more sugary food. Other people, however, seem less likely to gain weight if they eat only two meals a day (depending on what they are eating). Dietary requirements vary by body type and blood type. In the 1930s, William Sheldon, M.D., classified body types as "ectomorphic" (long and thin), "mesomorphic" (muscular), and "endomorphic" (soft and round). Dr. Sheldon suggested that the overweight endomorphs are more likely to have long (forty-foot) intestinal tracts. They gain weight easily because they absorb every calorie ingested. People of this body type fare better if they avoid calorie-dense foods like fats, sugar, and white-flour products. They also do well as vegetarians, and they particularly need exercise.

If your child refuses to eat anything but junk food, let him skip a meal. He won't starve, and when he is hungry enough, he'll eat vegetables. Don't serve dessert with every meal; save it for special occasions. Don't make dessert a reward for eating everything on his plate: You'll train him to force-feed, losing touch with his body's signals for its real nutritional needs. A better approach is to serve smaller portions of the entire meal, and allow a small portion of dessert for a child who *tries* everything on his plate. For other dietary suggestions, see "Nutrition."

For children who are underweight, alfalfa supplements can stimulate the appetite and help them put weight on.

PACIFIERS (See Nail Biting)

PAIN, INFLAMMATION

INFANTS AND young children will cry to let the world know things are not right, but finding and treating the cause is up to the parent, who must look for nonverbal clues. A pinched look about the eyes and a wrinkled forehead may mean a headache. A limp indicates trouble in the knee, hip, or ankle. Doubling up suggests abdominal pain. (See "Abdominal Pain.") If simple home measures don't work to pinpoint and relieve the crisis, a doctor's examination may be required.

 ### Pharmaceutical Pain Relief

ADULTS IN the habit of popping analgesics for their own aches and pains may approach their children's pain in the same way, but these drugs are more hazardous for children. Aspirin has been linked to an often fatal disease called Reye's syndrome when used in the treatment of childhood viral infections; and you may not know when your child is suffering from something in that category. (See "Fever," "Reye's Syndrome.") Aspirin also keeps blood platelets from sticking together normally, so avoid its use particularly for newborns and pregnant women. Acetaminophen (Tylenol, Datril, Anacin-3, Panadol, Liquiprin) has replaced aspirin as the analgesic of choice for children, but it, too, poses risks. Just ten Extra-Strength Tylenol can be fatal to a child, and even small overdoses of either aspirin or acetaminophen can be life-threatening. In large doses, acetaminophen can cause irreversible liver damage and death even in adults.[192]

Some pediatricians favor ibuprofen (Advil, PediaProfen, and others). Its side effects are similar to aspirin's, but their incidence may be lower. Adverse reactions with other drugs are less likely with ibuprofen, and overdosing is less likely to have serious consequences, but the drug still isn't harmless. To avoid an upset stomach, give it along with food. Ibuprofen isn't recommended for women who are pregnant or nursing, or for people who have stomach problems or are allergic to aspirin.

 ## Natural Alternatives

THE SAFEST pain relievers are homeopathic medicines. For reducing inflammation, Hypericum 30c can work as well as aspirin without the risk of side effects. Give three pills four times daily. For pain from injury, give Arnica. Hyland's makes a homeopathic headache formula good for occasional headache. Migramed by CompliMed is a good combination homeopathic remedy to try for your child's migraine headache. For other homeopathic remedies, see "Headaches," "Trauma," and "Surgical Trauma."

Herbal remedies are also effective. For migraine headaches, the herb feverfew has been touted as a miracle cure that can eliminate the need for drugs and their concomitant side effects; see "Headaches" for fuller discussion.

Some nutrients are also natural anti-inflammatories, which reduce pain either by decreasing local fluid levels or because of diuretic properties that reduce inflammation. They include vitamins C and B_6, potassium, and many herbs. Magnesium is another natural pain reliever. Too-low levels of magnesium increase nerve cell excitability and pain.[193]

Improving circulation can help relieve pain by eliminating pain-response chemicals and exhausted immune system cells. Effective therapies include massage, acupressure, heat treatments, stretching, and exercise.[194]

PARASITES (PINWORMS, AMOEBAS, INTESTINAL WORMS)

PARASITES ARE common in children, particularly if they suck their thumbs, which allows the eggs to be carried from hand to mouth. *Pinworms* are the most common type of parasite, troubling 80 percent of children sometime during childhood. Symptoms include night wakefulness, an itchy anal area, stomachaches, and general irritability from not sleeping well. A persistent dry cough may also be a sign of worms.

Other parasites that may infect children include *amoebas* and similar *intestinal worms*. The Centers for Disease Control now documents fifteen to twenty outbreaks of waterborne parasites each year in the United States. Experts speculate that the true number of outbreaks is in the hundreds, since parasitic illnesses are often mistaken for stomach flu and other intestinal disorders. A 1994 study put the hidden parasite epidemic at two million U.S. cases per year.[195] Symptoms of infestation include gas and bloating, irritable bowel syndrome, joint and muscle aches and pains, skin conditions, granulomas, nervousness, sleep disturbances, anemia, allergy, constipation, diarrhea, tooth grinding, chronic fatigue, and immune dysfunction.[196]

Giardia is a protozoan resident of the intestinal tracts of humans and animals. More people are infected with this parasite than is realized. The common assumption is that they must be violently ill and vomiting, but Giardia can also be living in the systems of apparently healthy people. Their immune systems are strong enough to keep it at bay, so they don't get seriously ill, but they may have vague abdominal complaints. The main symptoms are gas, bloating, abdominal discomfort, and alternating diarrhea and constipation. The symptom complex is compounded when the parasites and their host stress each other. When the host is stressed, the pH of the intestines drops, causing parasites to become more active and the person to feel more bloated and miserable; when the parasites living in the body get upset, the person gets more irritable, edgy, and emotional.

Trichinosis is an infection caused by a nematode (a worm), resulting from the ingestion of insufficiently cooked meat containing the encysted larvae of *T. spiralis*. The incidence of infection in humans has declined, but it is still sometimes found in people eating sausage made from uncooked pork. Diagnosis is made by a muscle biopsy showing the encapsulated larvae. To avoid parasitic infections of this sort, do not serve or eat partially cooked or uncooked meat or fish. Japanese sushi (raw fish) is a notorious carrier of parasitic infection.

Food poisoning is often confused with parasites or worms (see "Food Poisoning"), while conditions diagnosed as more serious intestinal diseases, like Crohn's disease or colitis, sometimes turn out to be simply parasitic infections.

 Drug Treatment

FOR PINWORMS, pediatricians typically prescribe mebendazole (Vermox). It kills the worms but must be repeated in ten days to kill the next generation before they mature and multiply; and even then it may not be effective.

Standard treatment for Giardia and other intestinal parasites is metronidazole (Flagyl). It is of limited effectiveness and can have troubling side effects, including convulsive seizures, numbness in the extremities, nausea and vomiting, headache, and intestinal distress. It is an expensive drug required by law to bear the warning "Carcinogenic in rodents. Avoid unnecessary use." To avoid giving metronidazole unnecessarily, testing for parasites is always prescribed in the U.S. before treatment; but stool tests are notoriously unreliable, so parasites often go undetected and untreated. **Caution: Metronidazole should not be combined with alcohol, even the alcohol in cough syrup.**

Home Diagnosis and Treatment of Pinworms

ADULT FEMALE pinworms come out at night to lay their eggs. They are a quarter inch long, white, and wiggly. To check for them, parents can sneak into the child's bedroom at night, pull down the covers, and shine a flashlight at the anal area. Or try the Scotch tape trick: If tape is put over the opening in a child's buttocks, the worms will stick to the tape and can be seen.

Another indicator involves the moon. Worms lay their eggs and are most active when the moon is full. If a child's symptoms are most pronounced at that time, he or she may have pinworms.

Pediatricians receive midnight calls every week from parents concerned that their children will be eaten up with pinworms if immediate action isn't taken. Although nothing actually has to be done immediately, you can try the garlic enema: Boil two garlic cloves in a quart of water, let the water cool, then let the fluid run in and out of the child's rectum. The procedure is facilitated by bringing a cushioned chair up to the tub and placing the child facedown on the chair, with his or her legs hanging into the tub.

Pinworms eliminated through bowel movements can be spread to others. To prevent reinfection from themselves or others, keep children's fingernails short and dirt-free and their underwear clean; and encourage them to stop sucking their fingers.

Natural Alternatives to Drugs

HOMEOPATHS MAINTAIN that drugs like Vermox and Flagyl don't actually kill parasites but merely push them deeper into the system. The patients keep coming back with worms, which are even harder to get rid of after the drugs have driven them deeper into the body. Symptoms of deeply suppressed pinworms include chronic dry cough, itchy bottom around the full moon, grinding teeth, and aggressive behavior (biting, pinching, etc.).

A homeopathic remedy called Cina is an effective, nontoxic alternative for eliminating pinworms permanently. The dosage is two pills three times a day of Cina 30x (or for more severe cases, Cina 200x) for four days. In some cases, it needs to be repeated every month for four days around the full moon for a full year to prevent worm reinfestation.

Other very effective homeopathic options for a variety of parasites are Worms by CompliMed and Ver by Deseret. These remedies could take up to six months to work. How well they work and how long they take depends on how deeply the worms have embedded into the system. Children may have to go through a year's treatment to eliminate a deeply embedded worm infestation. The remedies are also recommended for prevention when eating out frequently or traveling abroad (ten drops once a day throughout the trip), or for an adult or child who gets home from a trip or a meal at an exotic restaurant complaining of an upset stomach, diarrhea, or other parasite symptoms. If the parasites have been in the body awhile, the remedies will give only symptomatic relief, but they can be used for occasional stomach upset while other remedies have time to work.

Antiparasitic herbs include wormwood, black walnut, cloves, and valerian. They can be mixed and taken at a dosage of two droppersful three times daily in water mixed with a teaspoonful of Luvos Healing Earth. To rout parasites that have been in residence for some time, a four- to six-week course of treatment is generally necessary. The best protocol seems to be an herbal parasite combination developed by MarcoPharma that includes an antiparasitic remedy called Para A, an antimicrobial remedy, Luvos to heal lesions, and other remedial agents. Another herbal solution for a variety of parasites is Clarkia 100 by Bio-Nutritional Formulas.

Parasite-eliminating herbs used in Mexico and Central America include Apasote (pigweed) made into a soup and Jacaranda made into a tea.

For Giardia, the nondrug remedy that seems to be most effective is a Staufen homeopathic from Germany called Lamblia. Comparable series therapy is available in the United States from Deseret. The prescribed regimen is one ampule (containing varying potencies from 30x to 5x) every three days for one month.

Also good is a remedy called Giardia by Hanna Kroeger; however, it works only on newly acquired Giardia. The recommended dose is ten drops three times a day until the bottle is empty.

See also "Toxoplasmosis."

Pinworms Eliminated with Homeopathics after Drugs Failed

Nine-year-old Max had rectal itching at night, a dry cough that had lingered for months, and stomach pains. He also ground his teeth at night. His mother confirmed that he had had pinworms twice and had taken medication for them each time. When the mother checked with Scotch tape, she found that he still had pinworms. She reported that he also got more irritable and active around the full moon. Author Dr. Walker gave him Cina 200, beginning each month around the full moon. After about five months of this treatment, his mother called in amazement to say that his cough had gone away and he had begun sleeping better and doing better in school. He also looked healthier, quit biting his nails, quit grinding his teeth, and the black circles under his eyes went away.

PERTUSSIS (See Whooping Cough)

PHOBIAS (See Anxiety)

PICA

PICA, THE eating of nonfoods, is a giveaway clue that some mineral is missing in the diet or that the body is otherwise out of balance. Children and adults with iron-deficiency anemia may have an inclination to eat dirt or ice. Calcium and magnesium may be lacking as well. Pregnant women have been known to eat laundry starch or plaster off the wall looking for calcium, while a craving for chocolate may indicate a magnesium deficiency. A blood test can be given to determine mineral deficiencies, although they won't always be found. Homeopathic theory attributes pica to a vibrational imbalance in the body, the same type of imbalance that leads to cravings for sugar, salt, vinegar, or sour foods.

If iron-deficiency anemia is the problem, ferrous fumarate is the usual remedy. A pregnant woman craving nonfoods should make a trip to the health food store for some mineral supplements.

For a craving for chalk and other calcium-containing indigestibles, the homeopathic remedy is Calc carb. For other nonfood cravings, consult a homeopath.

PIGEON TOES

PIGEON TOES, or the tendency of the feet to turn inward, begins when the fetus wraps his feet around his stomach in the cramped uterus. This comfortable position is maintained if the infant sleeps on his stomach with his buttocks resting on the turned-in feet, a position that puts torsion on the tibial (shin) bone, causing it to spiral inward. Pigeon toes can be seen easily when the child is sitting with legs dangling. One should be able to draw a straight line from the kneecap to the second toe; in the pigeon-toed, the feet will turn in. Most children outgrow the condition as they get taller and sleep in different positions, especially on the side and back. If the problem makes the child stumble, however, a doctor may recommend orthopedic shoes to help the feet turn outward.

PINKEYE (See Eye Infection)

PINWORMS (See Parasites)

PLANTAR WARTS (See Warts)

PNEUMONIA

PNEUMONIA IS a term that includes a number of different conditions that infect or inflame the lungs, caused by a number of different agents. Bacteria and viruses are the most common, but fungi, mycoplasmas, and inhalants are other possibilities. Estimates are that more than four million cases of pneumonia occur annually in the United States. People considered at high risk include the very young, the elderly, and those with chronic underlying health problems. In very young children with immature immune systems, viral pneumonia is the most common form of the disease. Symptoms mimic the flu and include fever, dry cough, headache, muscle pain, weakness, and breathlessness. The more serious bacterial pneumonia, usually caused by pneumococcus bacteria, accounts for an estimated forty thousand deaths yearly. Symptoms in severe cases include shaking, chills, chattering teeth, severe chest pains, sweats, cough that produces rust-colored or greenish mucus, increased breathing and pulse rate, and a bluish tint to the lips or nails caused by lack of oxygen. Mycoplasmas (microorganisms that are smaller than bacteria and lack cell walls) are responsible for another 20 percent of cases of pneumonia.

Conventional Treatment

EARLY TREATMENT with antibiotics can eliminate the serious symptoms of bacterial pneumonia and can speed recovery from mycoplasma pneumonia; but there are no effective treatments for most types of viral pneumonia, since antibiotics don't work on viruses. Fortunately, viral pneumonia usually heals on its own.[197]

Natural Alternatives

HERBS CAN help the body with the healing process. The herbs elecampe and lungwort are particularly good. Another good herbal pneumonia remedy for children twelve and over is the Chinese formula Ping Chuan, which dries up excess fluid in the chest.

Homeopaths maintain that even for bacterial pneumonia, antibiotics do not eliminate the organisms that cause it; they merely push the invaders farther in. When the system is run-down and under stress, the condition returns. Only when the disease has been brought to the surface and eliminated can it be cured for good. Homeopathic remedies help stimulate this process, although the pneumonia victim who does not have a strong immune system may still require antibiotics if the condition is not caught early enough. If the patient is very run-down, recovery on herbs and homeopathic remedies will be slow, and he or she is likely to continue to get weaker in the meantime. If antibiotics are used, homeopathic remedies should still be taken, to prevent the pneumonia from returning year after year.

An excellent homeopathic remedy for clearing pneumonia from the system is a German formula by Staufen called Mixed Pneumonia;

comparable series therapy is available in the U.S. from Deseret. There is also a special homeopathic called Myco Pneumonia for mycoplasma pneumonia. Dulpulmon by CompliMed is a good combination homeopathic product. The dosage is ten drops every fifteen minutes to start, then four times daily as needed until well.

POISONING

POISONING IS common in children, who tend to investigate things by eating them. The contents of the purse on the counter are a mystery that must be investigated, often by mouth. Cleaning solutions, soaps, polishes, and drain cleaners seem to leap out at children and ask to be explored. All homes should have the phone number of the local Poison Control Center on hand, along with syrup of Ipecac for emergency use. When this drug is swallowed, the child usually vomits, typically emptying the stomach better than if it were pumped in a doctor's office. The Poison Control Center should be consulted before syrup of Ipecac is given, however, because some things shouldn't be vomited; vomiting petroleum distillates, for example, can be dangerous due to the chance of aspiration into the lungs. If circumstantial evidence points to ingestion of something toxic and the Poison Control Center approves, give the dose of Ipecac recommended on the label, then seat the child outdoors and wait for the coming explosion. Another option is in front of the toilet bowl, but distressed children are bad shots.

 Basic Poison Prevention

KEEP ALL medicines and supplements out of children's reach and in child-resistant containers with the lids on tight. Lock up medicines, and teach kids the difference between medicine and candy. If you praise them for taking medicine, caution them at the same time about its dangers. Don't take medicine in front of your child or give it to one child while another is watching. Always read label directions before giving a child medicine. Keep cleaning products, insect sprays, automobile products, paint products, fertilizers, and similar products out of children's reach and locked up. Lye products are extremely dangerous and should not be kept in the house.[198]

POISON IVY, POISON OAK (See Itching)

PREMENSTRUAL SYNDROME (PMS)

PREMENSTRUAL SYNDROME (PMS) is usually thought of as beginning sometime in the thirties, when hormone production is slowing down; but girls in their teens may also have premenstrual tension, with increased irritability, mood swings, and crying jags. PMS is a cluster of uncomfortable symptoms that sets in seven to ten days before menstruation begins, including headaches, abdominal bloating, breast swelling, fluid retention, increased thirst, increased appetite, cravings for sweet or salty foods, and emotional symptoms including anxiety, mood swings, depression, hostility, and loss of self-confidence.

PMS symptoms are due to a hormone imbalance before menstruation. During the normal menstrual cycle, immediately after ovulation, levels of both estrogen and progesterone rise, and they continue to rise until menstruation. The progesterone acts as an estrogen antagonist, keeping estrogen levels in check. But progesterone stores can be depleted by stress (emotional, dietary, or environmental), causing progesterone to be converted to the stress hormone cortisol. Without enough progesterone, estrogen levels get too high. Excess estrogen can then produce salt and fluid retention, low blood sugar, blood clotting, breast tenderness, thyroid problems, and weight gain. These physical imbalances produce the mood swings and other psychological effects associated with PMS.[199]

Conventional Treatment

MIDOL, A combination painkiller and diuretic (a "water pill" that increases the excretion of urine), is often recommended to relieve PMS. The problem is that diuretics work by forcing the kidneys to release body fluid; and with the excess water go important minerals and chemicals, throwing off electrolyte and mineral balance. That's why most diuretics are prescription-only drugs; in fact, PMS is the *only* condition for which their over-the-counter use is approved, and that is just because the pills are intended for use only a few days each month.

Natural Alternatives

CHINESE AND homeopathic doctors believe in aiding the body to produce and balance its own hormones. Chinese medicine attributes PMS to a congested liver. The diet of teenage girls today tends to be junk-food rich, laden with sugar, food coloring, and preservatives. These toxins need to be broken down by the liver along with the monthly hormone load. When the liver gets congested, it has trouble clearing hormones properly and they get out of balance in the body. Green vegetables, chlorophyll, and nutritional products like Ultimate Green can help clean the liver. See "Environmental Illness."

Relaxed Wanderer, the brand name for a Chinese patent formula called Hsiao Yao Wan (or Xiao Yao Tang), is an excellent remedy for PMS. It works particularly well for those with a tendency to be cold (especially the hands and feet).

Homeopathic remedies are also available for treating PMS. Natural Phases by Boiron effectively relieves moodiness and irritability in teens. Pulsatilla is also good for teenage girls who are emotional and experience mood swings.

To relieve edema or bloating, a clinical study showed that dandelion leaf works as well as Lasix, a popular diuretic. Parsley is another option. MarcoPharma makes an asparagus concentrate that is a good diuretic. A homeopathic option is Mededema by CompliMed. Drinking less and avoiding salt and salt-rich foods that cause water retention can also help.

The hormone imbalance on which PMS has been blamed may be the result of nutritional imbalances. Studies show that women on high-fiber, low-fat diets have less PMS, less breast cancer, less premenstrual breast pain, and less trouble with their menstrual periods.[200] Calcium can also help relieve PMS symptoms.[201] Other nutritional supplements shown to help include vitamins B_6 and E, and essential fatty acids (evening primrose oil, black currant oil, borage). Avoidance of caffeine and allergenic foods may also help.[202] So may natural progesterone cream (Pro-Gest), made from a type of Mexican yam. For more detailed information, see Ellen Brown and Lynne Walker, *Menopause and Estrogen* (1996).

PSORIASIS (See Dermatitis)

PUBERTY IN GIRLS (See Menstrual Problems)

PULSE

THE PULSE, or number of heartbeats per minute, is usually between 80 and 100 in children. A too-rapid heartbeat may indicate a defect in the nerve conduction fibers in the heart. A pediatrician should address this problem.

RABIES (See Animal Bites)

RASH (See Itching, Diaper Rash)

REYE'S SYNDROME

REYE'S SYNDROME is a complex of muscle inflammation and neurological symptoms that normally develops several days after a viral infection—flu, chicken pox, or a cold. Though uncommon, the condition is usually fatal; and among those who survive, about 15 percent suffer from mental retardation, paralysis, or other neurological disorders. The course of the illness is rapid. The young child appears to have a minor cold but soon experiences vomiting, headache, and lethargy. In a day or two, coma develops and death usually follows, apparently from swollen brain tissue from fat infiltration occurring in the liver and brain (cerebral edema). Symptoms to watch for are persistent vomiting, listlessness, drowsiness, personality changes, disorientation, delirium, convulsions, or loss of consciousness. Treatment, however, is normally too late to be effective.

Reye's syndrome has now been linked to aspirin taken to reduce fever and headache during a viral infection. The National Reye's Syndrome Foundation (NRSF), the U.S. Surgeon General, the Food and Drug Administration, the Centers for Disease Control, and the American Academy of Pediatrics recommend that aspirin and combination products containing aspirin not be taken by anyone under nineteen years of age during fever-causing illnesses.

Bayer, Anacin, Excedrin, and other popular painkillers now come in aspirin-free forms. For natural analgesic alternatives, see "Fever," "Pain," "Headaches."

RHEUMATIC FEVER (See Strep Throat)

RHINITIS (RUNNY NOSE), SINUSITIS

RHINITIS (A runny nose) is usually caused by a virus, but hay fever or allergies will also show watery discharge. (See "Colds," "Allergies.") A viral cold generally lasts seven days.

If the nasal discharge becomes cloudy, green, or yellow, a secondary bacterial infection is indicated. A bacterial infection is usually responsible for *sinusitis,* or inflammation of the sinuses. The sinuses are airfilled cavities lined with mucous membranes above and below the eyes. Sinusitis is characterized by persistent nasal congestion, cold or flulike symptoms that go beyond the usual seven to ten days, and pain and headache in the sinus area. People who are particularly susceptible to sinusitis are those with allergies or deformities of the nose (such as a deviated septum) and those habitually exposed to bacteria.

Sinusitis is often confused with *allergic rhinitis,* which has similar symptoms but is not caused by bacteria. Besides environmental allergens (as in hay fever), allergic rhinitis may be caused by extreme temperature changes or overuse of nasal sprays.

 Conventional Treatment

DECONGESTANTS ARE often used for runny noses, but the drugs have side effects and can lead to a rebound effect, causing greater congestion and the need for more nasal spray when they wear off. (See "Colds.")

Antibiotics may be used for sinusitis, or for secondary bacterial infection in rhinitis; but an increasing number of cases of sinusitis are resistant to standard antibiotics like amoxicillin. Doctors have therefore resorted to other, more powerful and expensive antibiotics, or to a four- to six-week course of treatment with amoxicillin combined with Flagyl (metronidazole), a drug with substantial side effects of its own. (See

"Parasites.") Sinusitis that does not respond after several weeks of anti-biotic treatment is termed chronic and is referred to a specialist. When antibiotics don't work, surgery may be the next resort.

For allergic rhinitis, which isn't caused by bacteria, antibiotics are not effective. The condition is treated conventionally with antihistamines and decongestants. If those drugs don't work, corticosteroids are gener-ally prescribed. (See "Allergies.")

Caution: If over-the-counter decongestant nose drops or sprays containing phenylephrine (for example, Neo-Synephrine) are resorted to, they should not be continued for more than three days, since they can cause addiction.

 Homeopathic Treatment

HOMEOPATHS USE remedies that encourage rather than prevent the nose from running, in order to clear out old infections permanently. In fact, homeopaths consider drugs that stop the nose from running to be a principle *cause* of sinus infections. When drainage is stopped, bacte-ria are trapped in the nose, where they fester and produce infection. Antibiotics taken for a sinus infection do not actually "kill" these bacte-ria but merely push the germs farther into the sinuses. The symptoms go away temporarily, but they recur when the body tries to push the bacteria out again.

If homeopathic treatment is accompanied at the first sign of a sinus problem by procedures to drain the lymph glands, infection can usually be stopped before it starts. Lymph-draining procedures include mas-sage to stimulate the lymph glands, drinking substantial amounts of water (a large glass every hour), lymphatic and bouncing exercises to move the lymph, and lymph-draining homeopathic remedies. Particu-larly good are Lymphomyosot by Heel and Lymphonest by Nestmann. (The latter has a strong herbal taste and requires dilution in water for children.) The throat can be cleared of mucus by gargling with warm water. For older children, a *neti* pot (an Indian device available from yoga centers and the Internet) may be used to flush the sinuses. The flow of mucus can be stimulated by having the patient lie on his or her back, then applying hot and cold compresses to the forehead and cheeks. Increase humidity, especially in bedrooms.

For chronic sinusitis, a German homeopathic remedy called Peptostrep, taken in strengths ranging from 200x to 5x over a period of a month, is remarkably effective in clearing sinusitis for good. It makes the nose run and pushes out old infection. Problems generally occur only if the sufferer resorts to drugs that stop the cleansing, putting him back where he started. An equivalent American homeopathic remedy is available from Deseret.

For younger children, homeopathic remedies are best; but for older children, you can try herbal remedies. One good for relieving rhinitis, sinusitis, and bronchitis is a gemmotherapy by Dolisos called European Filbert.

Chinese patent herbal remedies that are effective in treating sinusitis in children thirteen and older include Pe Min Kan Wan and Be Yin Lin. For both, the recommended dosage is two to three pills two to three times daily.

Western herbal products good for treating the condition include Sinuplex by Metagenics and Decongest Herbal by Zand.

For other natural remedies useful for treating runny noses, see "Colds."

RIB FRACTURES (See Bones, Broken or Fractured)

RICKETS (See Sunburn)

RINGWORM (See Fungal Infections)

ROSEOLA (See Measles)

RUBELLA/GERMAN MEASLES (See Measles)

SALMONELLA (See Food Poisoning)

SCABIES

SCABIES (SOMETIMES called the seven-year itch) is a contagious skin disease caused by mites. The mother mite burrows under the thin layers of skin of the wrists, webs of the fingers, groin, armpits, and genitalia. Eggs are then laid in these burrows, setting up an intense, unignorable itch. Impetigo is a common secondary infection. (See "Impetigo.")

 Conventional Treatment

THE DRUG recommended by the American Academy of Pediatrics is 5 percent permethrin. Possible side effects include burning, stinging, numbness, pain, and rash. Lindane is also suggested, but it is a toxic drug that must be used cautiously. (See "Head Lice.")

 Natural Alternative Treatment

TEA TREE oil is an effective nontoxic alternative. Apply over the whole affected area twice a day for three to four days. Other herbal options include Balsam of Peru, comfrey-root topical salve, and Calendula and goldenseal ointments.

Homeopathic remedies for scabies include Antimonium crudum (for dry skin rash with pimples; itching worse at night), Arsenicum album (for a dry, rough, scaly rash; rash worse with exposure to cold; itching may be accompanied by burning sensation or restlessness), and sulphur (for the child who is sweaty, with red, dry, hot-looking skin patches).[203]

Homeopaths consider scabies indicative of a miasm (roughly equivalent to a genetic tendency) that can lead to psoriasis later in life. To treat this "psora" miasm, see a homeopath.

SCARS (See Dermatitis)

SCOLIOSIS

Scoliosis is a curving of the spine to one side. Its cause is unknown. Not uncommonly, adolescent girls develop the condition during the growth spurt associated with the onset of puberty. Scoliosis is easily diagnosed if checked, but it is not painful and therefore may be overlooked until its advanced stages. An alert mother may observe, however, that her daughter holds one hip noticeably higher than the other, or the doctor may find some asymmetry in the girl's back during a routine physical. X rays show the extent of the curve.

 Conventional Treatment

If the child has not reached her adult height, an elaborate brace may be imposed from chin to hips, which can partially correct the bend to an acceptable position. If that doesn't work, a cast may be used to hold it. Some orthopedic surgeons will use special metal rods secured to the vertebrae to arrest the process.

Alternative Treatment

BEFORE SUBMITTING your child to these drastic procedures, try body-work: chiropractic, craniosacral adjustment, Zero Balancing, or Pilates. Miracle cures have been reported that not only avoid painful invasive surgery and restrictive casts but strengthen and rebalance the whole body.

Scoliosis Corrected without Braces or Surgery

Mrs. Lauralee Bruce of Long Island was diagnosed with scoliosis in her teens. Her doctor intended to fuse her joints and insert a metal rod in her back. Instead, she did Pilates training and has been fine ever since. At forty-eight, she has been a Pilates instructor for twenty years and still has the figure of a young woman. She may be reached for consultation at 631-725-7995 or 631-725-5774.

SEIZURES, EPILEPSY, CONVULSIONS

SEIZURES CAN range from mild to severe and may be triggered by epilepsy, fever, magnesium deficiency, electrolyte imbalances (excess alkalinity), and hypoglycemia, among other initiators. Children prone to them may outgrow them with age.

The milder form of seizure, the "petit mal," consists of momentary staring into space without loss of muscular control. These seizures can occur without the sufferer or the people nearby even realizing it; some seizures show only as alterations of thoughts or feelings. The "grand mal" seizure is the violent form in which the victim cries out, falls down, stiffens throughout the body, and shakes all over. Eventually he or she relaxes, and calmness and often sleep follow.

Epilepsy is sudden abnormal electrical activity of the brain that leads to repeated seizures or convulsions (violent involuntary contractions of the voluntary muscles). The EEG (electroencephalogram or brain-wave test) is the usual diagnostic indicator. Epilepsy typically shows as an "irritable focus" in the cortex of the brain, which initiates the erratic nervous system activity that then spreads to other parts of the brain. If the motor area is involved, the muscles are also affected.

Febrile seizures are seizures triggered by fever (see "Fever"). Parents tend to panic when their child has one of these episodes, which can appear quite alarming; but most seizures stop in a few minutes and don't cause long-term harm. The parent needs only to remain calm, check the clock, and make sure the child is lying down on his side in a safe place away from sharp objects. If the seizure lasts more than four minutes, call 911 (the emergency hotline) or take the child to the nearest emergency room. If it lasts less than four minutes, you can take him to either your regular pediatrician or the emergency room. Don't try to put anything in his mouth to prevent swallowing his tongue, which isn't actually a threat.[204]

 ## Conventional Treatment

DRUGS ARE used to control seizures, including phenytoin (Dilantin), phenobarbital, and tegretol. They are necessary to prevent damage to the brain and body, but none stops convulsions completely, and side effects are common, including drowsiness and irritability.

 ## Alternative Treatment

HOMEOPATHIC REMEDIES can help correct imbalances in the body. Young girls may develop seizures when they begin menstruating. The homeopathic remedy for this is Bufo 200c. For seizures caused by concussion of the brain (head injury), the remedy is Circuta. For jerking, twitching, and trembling of the limbs or sudden inward jerking of the fingers caused by worms, the remedy is Cina 200c. For epileptic seizures beginning in the fingers, palms, and toes, the remedy is Cuprum metallicum. Consult a constitutional homeopath for the appropriate remedy and dose.

Certain nutrients are also thought to be of benefit, including selenium, manganese, GABA, and vitamin B_6. Seizures can be caused by a sodium imbalance in the blood, in which case vinegar may help, as it removes sodium from the system. Give one teaspoonful of apple cider vinegar in an eight-ounce glass of water. If the child likes the taste, he probably needs it; children's tastebuds are still sensitive enough to be

Seizures Eased with Natural Remedy

A girl who began having repeated seizures was brought by her mother to see author Dr. Walker. The seizures had gotten longer and more frequent; the girl was having them every few days for eight to ten minutes at a time. The mother was concerned about putting her daughter on medication and was looking for alternative options. Dr. Walker told the mother she could not recommend alternative treatment for legal reasons, but she could recommend natural remedies to increase the girl's vital life force and balance her subtle energies, which might indirectly help relieve the seizures. The girl's history indicated she was a classic case for the homeopathic remedy Tarentula hispanica (a constitutional remedy specific for this child). After the remedy was given, the girl had only two more seizures, which were a month apart, lasted less than a minute each, and barely involved loss of consciousness. The condition then disappeared completely.

responsive to the body's needs. Give this remedy three times a day until it begins to taste too sour, when the dose can be lowered to once every day or two.

One epilepsy sufferer whose seizures were not controlled by drugs alone reported gaining control by using a mixture of herbs including damiana, gotu kola, Siberian ginseng, skullcap, St.-John's-wort, and ginkgo biloba.

SHOCK, FAINTING, EMOTIONAL TRAUMA

SHOCK INVOLVES blood pressure low enough to prevent oxygenation of body tissues, particularly the brain. It can have a variety of causes, including septicemia (blood poisoning), anaphylaxis (an exaggerated allergic reaction to injection of a foreign protein), an allergic reaction to a bee sting, electric shock, and blood volume depletion by prolonged vomiting and diarrhea. Call 911 (the emergency hotline) immediately in these cases and keep the patient prone. In the event of bleeding, apply pressure by hand; it's safer than a tourniquet. Comfort and reassurance are important, but extra warmth is not indicated. Fainting is a mild form of shock, but one that is easily treated by keeping the patient in a recumbent position (lying down).

 Natural Remedies

HOMEOPATHIC REMEDIES can help in cases of shock. For mental or emotional shock or trauma, the remedy is Aconite in a high potency. For physical trauma, the remedy is Arnica in a high potency. For electric shock, the remedy is Electricity 200x.

For shock from a bee sting, the hospital will give antihistamines and steroids (see "Insect Bites"), but homeopathic Apis may be administered in the meantime.

For anaphylactic shock from a vaccine reaction, call the doctor or hospital immediately. Homeopathic remedies can help relieve the crisis in the interim. Thuja helps counteract an allergic reaction to vaccines. Silicea is another option. Some homeopaths give homeopathic Sulphur to a child whose skin gets red and swollen at the site of an injection or who appears to be going into shock. CompliMed makes a remedy called Vaccinations that is good for relieving the effects of a vaccine received in the past (see "Immunizations").

For emotional trauma and to calm the nerves, Rescue Remedy, a Bach flower remedy, is effective and completely safe.

Vaccine Reaction Relieved with a Homeopathic Remedy

Jenny, who works in a pharmacy, reports this case: A mother came in with her six-month-old daughter just to shop. While the mother and Jenny were talking, the child started looking distressed, then turning blue. The mother told Jenny the baby had just received her infant immunizations. Jenny rushed to get some Silicea, but before she could get the bottle open, the baby began having seizures. As soon as Jenny placed the remedy in the baby's mouth, the seizures stopped and her color returned to normal. The mother called later to say the baby was fine. Jenny believes that if she had not given Silicea, the baby may have died.

SINUSITIS (See Rhinitis)

SKIN CANCER (See Sunburn)

SKIN INFECTIONS: ABSCESSES, BOILS, CARBUNCLES, FOLLICULITIS; INFECTIONS FROM SPLINTERS, CACTUS BURRS, BODY PIERCINGS

AN *ABSCESS* is a collection of pus caused by a skin infection. The ordinary (or pyogenic) abscess may be found in any tissue of the body—in the center of bone, in the appendix, in the lymph glands, in infected gum tissue around the teeth, etc. For all pyogenic abscesses located near the surface of the body, the symptoms are the same: pain, tenderness, and a mass with a red, firm surface and soft center. The temperature and white blood count are usually elevated. A *cold abscess* is a nontender swelling without fever.

Boils and *carbuncles* are quite painful localized abscesses that form in the skin and underlying tissues, usually as a result of infection that has gained entry by traveling down into the hair follicles.

Folliculitis is the presence of pustules in the hair follicles.

Other skin infections may result from surface wounds to the body, as from *splinters* and *cactus burrs*. A modern source of infection is the decorative *body piercing* that is increasingly popular among teenagers.

For impetigo, a contagious infection of the skin, see "Impetigo." For dental abscesses, see "Dental Problems."

 Conventional Treatment

PYOGENIC ABSCESSES containing pus are opened and drained, usually under general anesthesia. Carbuncles and boils are also opened if pus is demonstrated, but cold abscesses are aspirated (removed by suction), since there is a danger of secondary infection if they are opened. To rout infection in these and other abscesses, antibiotics are usually prescribed.

Natural Alternatives

THE PROBLEM with treating boils and carbuncles with antibiotics is that the abscesses are liable to recur and may take months for resolution. Folliculitis also tends to recur when treated with antibiotics and can lead to abscess formation. Homeopathic remedies can resolve these conditions permanently. The best single remedies are:

* Hepar sulph 30x: for the pus-forming abscess that is tender to the slightest touch, producing stabbing pain and irritability

* Silicea 6x: for the slow-forming abscess that is deep and will not go away or come to a head

* Pyrogenium 6c: for the deep infection with pus; or for "rotting flesh" (necrotic tissue that turns black from an insufficient supply of blood)

* Belladonna 30x: for the early-stage abscess that is red, hot, inflamed, and tender

* Gunpowder 8x: for folliculitis

Bacticin by CompliMed, a general remedy good for any type of infection, is the best combination homeopathic remedy available for abscesses. When it is used in place of antibiotics, you won't usually need prescription drugs. The dosage is ten drops every two hours the first day, then four times daily until cleared.

For infection from splinters or cactus burrs, herbal Black Ointment by Nature's Way will help draw out the infection.

Herbs can also help prevent folliculitis. Everyone has bacteria on the skin; but as with acne, not everyone gets folliculitis. Herbalists say the problem is caused by a reaction between the bacteria and toxins in the blood. Herbs can clear these toxins, preventing them from coming out in the hair follicles. Burdock taken internally cleans the blood and acts as a blood purifier. Other useful herbs are dandelion, echinacea, and slippery elm. Tea tree oil applied topically can also help clear folliculitis.

For boils, the infection can be brought to a head and readied for drainage (old-time doctors called it "laudable pus") using a hot, wet pack. Dissolve a teaspoon of salt (to keep the skin from becoming overly wrinkled) into a quart of hot water, then soak a hand towel in it. Wring out the towel and place it on the boil or infected area. Cover with plastic wrap and place a large, dry towel over that. Hold in place with an Ace bandage, tape, or pins. Leave this on for twelve hours or overnight. The effect is to keep heat and moisture on the affected area constantly. When the area is uncovered, it should be softer, cooler, less red, and less tender. Repeat the whole process if necessary.

For infection resulting from body piercing, wash with homeopathic Calendula mother tincture to clear up the infected area and promote healing. Infection can also be inhibited in its early stages with homeopathic Gunpowder 6x. Use the recommended dosage every two hours on the first day, then four times daily. The infection usually clears in two days.

For inflammation caused by an allergic reaction to the base metal in jewelry, switching to gold or silver should help.

SKIN RASH (See Dermatitis, Diaper Rash)

SORE THROAT (See Colds, Strep Throat)

SPEECH DEVELOPMENT, STUTTERING

SPEECH DEVELOPS slowly over the first few years of life. Delayed speech development is most commonly due to impaired hearing. If a child cannot hear the words, she cannot imitate them. One clue to this problem is that the child watches people's mouths instead of their eyes when they speak. A hearing test can pinpoint this problem. Pediatricians now have tests to check hearing in the newborn infant. See "Hearing Impairment."

Stuttering is common at about three years of age. One theory is that the child is trying to imitate the rapid speech of the parents. Children will normally outgrow this trait. Parents should avoid making comments about it in the meantime, which will merely make the child self-conscious and may cause stuttering to become a fixed habit.

SPRAINS

ANKLE SPRAINS are usually due to stepping on the outside of the foot, thereby pulling, stretching, or tearing the tendons that support the ankle joint. Other joints can also be sprained, including the wrists, fingers, and knees.

 Conventional Treatment

THE USUAL medical protocol is to use aspirin for pain and, in the case of ankle sprains, to use crutches to keep weight off the joint, typically for ten days. X rays are not usually necessary, but your doctor should make this determination.

 Alternative Treatment

SPRAINED JOINTS have been known to heal with remarkable speed using this combination approach:

1. Give the homeopathic remedy Trauma by CompliMed or Traumeel by BHI, ten drops orally every fifteen minutes for one hour, then ten drops every hour for four hours, then four times daily. These remedies also come as creams or ointments.

2. Apply the Chinese patent formula Tieh Ta Wan to the sprained ankle or injury. The remedy comes as a waxed ball containing an herbal paste wrapped in cellophane. Open the ball, remove the paste, add a few drops of water, and heat to a smooth consistency. Paint the ankle or injury with the paste, cover it, and keep it covered for twenty-four hours.

To further promote healing, try applying magnets to the acupuncture points above and below the injury. This technique is one used by acupuncturists to reestablish energy flow to the area.

In some cases, chiropractic adjustment has also brought immediate relief.

STAGE FRIGHT, NERVOUSNESS

NERVOUSNESS CAN ruin an artistic performance or a speech. Stage fright is distinguishable from chronic anxiety in that it goes away when the performance is over. Drugs like Valium may be used for stage fright, but they inhibit performance, cause side effects, and aren't recommended for young people.

 Natural Alternatives

HOMEOPATHIC REMEDIES can overcome stage fright without side effects. Gelsenium acts by retuning the emotions on a vibrational level. The child may take three pills every couple of hours before the speech or performance, then sip water in which several pellets have been dissolved during the event. Gelsenium also comes as a liquid that can be added to water. Another effective homeopathic option is a combination remedy called Nervousness by Natra-Bio.

Rescue Remedy, a Bach flower remedy, is also excellent for calming the nerves. Several drops in half a glass of water can be sipped while speaking or performing.

For children who blush or embarrass easily, Ambra grisea can be a face saver.

Flawless Performance with Homeopathics

Sixteen-year-old Jamie was so terrified at the rehearsal for her piano recital that she could not hold her hands steady on the keys. She took Nervousness, fifteen drops hourly for several hours before the performance. At the recital, she played her complicated piece flawlessly.

STOMACHACHE, INDIGESTION, BLOATING, GAS

CHILDREN OFTEN complain of stomachaches; but if they are not pale, vomiting, or feverish, you can usually allow the condition to pass without medical intervention. Natural remedies may be given at home to relieve symptoms. For remedies for stomachache with fever and vomiting, see "Intestinal Flu." For infant stomachaches, see "Colic."

If stomachaches are recurring, you need to try to track the cause. Many recurring stomachaches in children are related to food sensitivities. Likely culprits include cow's milk, wheat, corn, nuts, eggs, and citrus. Indigestion, bloating, cramps, and gas pains may also be traceable to wrong food combinations or to overeating. Children may have insufficient digestive enzymes to handle beans, cabbage, and other hard-to-digest foods, especially if ingested along with dairy, corn, wheat, or nuts. Indigestion can also be caused by drugs, including antihistamines, over-the-counter drugs, and antibiotics.

Stomachaches may also be attributable to ingestion of something toxic found in Grandmother's purse, under the sink, or in the medicine cabinet. Syrup of Ipecac, a powerful emetic, should be kept handy for these emergencies. Do not administer it, however, without first checking with the local Poison Control Center, since some poisonous substances should not be vomited. (See "Poisoning.") If circumstantial evidence points to ingestion of something toxic and the Poison Control Center approves, give the dose of Ipecac recommended on the label, then seat the child outdoors or in front of the toilet bowl and wait for the remedy to work.

Parasites can also cause stomachaches. Children are prone to picking up intestinal worms. Other symptoms include grinding the teeth, restless sleep, pain around the navel, restless behavior, pinching, and biting. All of these symptoms tend to get worse around the full moon, when intestinal worms lay their eggs. (See "Parasites," "Abdominal Pain.")

Other stomachaches may be traced to stress or anxiety over school or peer-group issues. One girl got diarrhea and an upset stomach every time she had a horseback-riding lesson. She wanted to be able to ride like her friends but was afraid of the horses. Another girl got a headache and upset stomach whenever she got ready for school. She later acknowledged that she was terrified of a certain teacher.

Over-the-Counter Drug Treatment for Indigestion

FOR STOMACHACHES caused by food, parents are liable to turn to antacids; but most of the advertised remedies for indigestion are meant for adults and can have harmful side effects, particularly if used repeatedly. Their cumulative effects can imbalance the body chemistry, making it too acidic or too alkaline.

Children as well as adults may feel uncomfortably bloated and distended after eating, but studies show that this feeling is *not* caused by excess gas, and the FDA has found no over-the-counter drugs that are safe or effective for alleviating it, TV ads notwithstanding.[205]

Natural Remedies for Indigestion

AT ONE time, pediatricians had mothers give their children cornstarch enemas to soothe the gut. This procedure usually silenced the child's complaints, though whether it was because the remedy worked or the cure was dreaded more than the ailment is hard to say. Enemas are no longer in fashion, but the principle was viable. Enemas addressed the cause rather than merely suppressing symptoms.

If the cause of recurring upset stomachs is a sensitivity to some food or foods, you need to find the triggers. Try systematically eliminating suspects. If the child suffered from colic as a baby, milk is high on the list. Other common offenders include wheat, eggs, nuts, sugar, and corn. (See "Allergies.") Also eliminate spicy foods, since young digestive systems aren't used to them.

Specific food sensitivities may also underlie the feeling of bloating and distention after eating. Excess belching has been traced to air swallowing. Stomach gas consists primarily of oxygen and nitrogen, which come from swallowed air. Increased air swallowing can be caused by eating rapidly, gulping, stress, gum chewing, thumb sucking, postnasal drip, dry mouth, or carbonated soft drinks.

If the cause of an upset stomach is emotional, Bach flower remedies can help. Rescue Remedy is one that has universal application.

A gemmotherapy good for upset stomachs is Fig Tree.

An essential oil good for stomachaches is peppermint oil. Place one drop in warm water and have the child drink it.

Herbs and herbal teas also offer safe and effective natural alternatives for settling the stomach, including licorice, ginger, peppermint, chamomile, and St.-John's-wort. Herbs for Kids makes Minty Ginger herbal drops to soothe an upset stomach. The recommended dosages are on the bottle.

Other good options for stomach complaints are Friendly Flora/Bifidus by Child Life and Rhino Tum-eez (wintergreen flavor) by Nutrition Now. Nutrition Now also makes a chewable raspberry-flavored acidophilus tablet that contains no dairy or whey, along with a powdered acidophilus product for children.

A good homeopathic remedy for simple indigestion with gas and bloating is Carbo Veg 6c. The recommended dosage is three tablets every fifteen minutes; for severe upset, give up to six doses. Also good are a combination product called Nux Vomica and Carbo Veg by Standard Homeopathic (give as needed every fifteen minutes after a meal, up to three doses) and Gastrica by CompliMed (five drops three times daily).

For intestinal gas, try homeopathic Ver by Deseret, Worms by CompliMed, or Gasalia by Boiron. Peppermint tea is an herbal remedy good for gas, bloating, and overeating.

Individual homeopathic remedies that can be quite effective for specific stomach symptoms include:

Arsenicum: if the child is pale, nervous, and vomiting from no known cause

Belladonna: if the child is very hot and restless

Mercuris: if the child is holding the stomach and looking uncomfortable (this remedy is actually for food poisoning)

Oscillococcinum: for flu symptoms

Recurring Vomiting Relieved with Homeopathic Remedy

A four-year-old boy who accompanied his musician father on the road began vomiting and got pale and nervous each night at the hotel. Although the cause wasn't determined, the syndrome appeared to have a psychological element. Arsenicum (three pills every half hour for three doses) relieved the problem.

STREP THROAT, RHEUMATIC FEVER

STREP THROAT is a sore throat due to streptococcal infection. It is usually a self-limited disease, meaning it will go away by itself without treatment.[206] The concern is that if it's left untreated, it can turn into rheumatic fever, a disease characterized by joint aches, fever, and heart murmurs. Deaths from rheumatic fever were once a serious threat, but today they are very rare in the United States. By 1970 they had plunged to about one per million.[207]

 Drug Treatment

DESPITE THIS dramatic decline in rheumatic fever, antibiotics are still routinely used in the treatment of strep throat to keep it from progressing. The downside is that the drugs themselves can be hazardous, resulting in allergic and toxic reactions and in "superinfections" by antibiotic-resistant organisms; and antibiotics are becoming less and less effective. The drugs also prevent the development of antibodies that defend against the disease. The child or adult who uses them is therefore liable to go through the winter with one sore throat after another. Given these risks and limited benefits, the prudent doctor should wait for a positive strep culture before initiating drug treatment. The odds that your child's painfully sore throat is caused by strep are less than one in five, and the odds that rheumatic fever will develop from it are about two in a million.

Caution: Once antibiotics are started, finish the full course even if test results later come back negative, to prevent any surviving bacteria from adapting to the drug and breeding antibiotic-resistant "superbugs."

 The Alternative Approach

EFFECTIVE HERBAL and homeopathic remedies are available. At the onset of a throat infection, give goldenseal and elderberry extract. Olive-leaf extract is another safe antibacterial and antiviral remedy. (See "Immunity.")

Chinese patent formulas are also available for treating strep throat and ordinary sore throats. Lu-Shen-Wan, when given for a very sore throat with fever, has been known to cure the condition in a single day. Zhong Gan Ling is effective for strep throat and sore throat with high fever and body aches. Fever is the distinguishing trait for this remedy.

If antibiotics are given, they will wipe out friendly along with unfriendly bacteria in the gut, paving the way for fungal overgrowth with *Candida albicans.* To aid recolonization with friendly flora, give acidophilus liquid or pills (two pills three times daily or as directed on the label) for two weeks between meals. Child Life makes Friendly Flora/Bifidus for kids. Nutrition Now makes a chewable raspberry-flavored acidophilus tablet that contains no dairy or whey, along with a powdered acidophilus product for children.

Among homeopathic remedies, the most effective for strep throat is a German Staufen remedy called Strep. Comparable series therapy is available in the United States from Deseret.

For other natural remedies for sore throats, see "Colds."

Strep Throat Cycle Broken

Eric, age eight, had had strep throat several times a year since he was five. The condition was so routine that his mother would simply telephone the doctor, who would then telephone the pharmacy with a prescription for another round of antibiotics. But the mother was concerned that the drugs weren't doing much good, and she wanted to break this cycle. Author Dr. Walker gave Eric the German Strep homeopathic formulation, along with acidophilus to reverse the harmful effects of repeated courses of antibiotics on his beneficial intestinal flora. Other remedies were used to build up his immune system.

It took some time for Eric to fully recover from his three years of being ill. First the suppressed bacteria had to surface, then the negative effects of the antibiotics had to be reversed, then his immune system had to build back up. When the suppressed germs started coming out, Eric seemed to be getting sick, but his mother understood the meaning of this healing crisis and persisted. (See Introduction.) After a few days of homeopathic treatment, Eric was clearly getting better; and after three months, he was quite well. Two years later, his mother reported that he had not been sick since he began the treatment.

STRESS

A LITTLE stress is a healthy motivator, but heavy stresses can do physical and emotional harm to children. Stress has become a way of life not only for adults but for children, whose overly busy schedules leave little time for daydreaming and playing in the grass. Particularly stressful situations include moving and changing schools, parental separation or divorce, violence or frequent arguing in the home, and being pushed to overachieve. Behavioral signs of stress include reverting to earlier habits like thumb sucking or bed-wetting, nightmares and other sleep disorders, hyperactivity, crying, withdrawal, moodiness, alcohol and drug abuse among teenagers, and lowered school performance. Physical effects include lowered immunity, more frequent colds, stomach ailments, headaches, eating too little or too much, and worsening of chronic conditions like asthma and diabetes.[208]

 Parental Relief

PARENTS CAN help by giving their stressed children emotional support and easing stresses at home. Parents often don't realize that the barrage of music lessons, dance lessons, foreign-language classes, after-school sports, and other extracurricular activities can be too much for children already pressured to achieve academically. Trying hard to please their parents, the children end up stressed. There are natural remedies that can help relieve the psychological sense of stress, but the first and most important step is to lighten the child's load and ease up on parental expectations. Let your child know he or she is loved unconditionally, without regard to performance.

Natural Remedies

BACH FLOWER remedies give excellent stress relief without side effects. Rescue Remedy is the universal option for children. Walnut is another remedy that is particularly good for times of change, as when moving to a new school or a new house, or when another child comes into the family.

Skullcap Oats by Eclectic Institute is an herbal remedy that calms children and allows them to get a good night's sleep. Another herbal remedy good for stress or tension is a gemmotherapy by Dolisos called Black Currant.

Aromatherapy is also calming and relaxing. Chamomile oil is good for the child who has trouble relaxing or is hyperactive, nervous, or upset. Put lavender oil in the bedroom, by or on the child's pillow or on a rag placed near the bed, or burn a lavender-scented candle in the room. Pillows are also made with lavender seeds in them.

Some children may be upset due to low blood sugar, which can set stress hormones racing. The safest and most natural treatment for hypoglycemia is to add magnesium and vitamin C to an optimal diet without sugar or junk food, and encourage the child to eat every two to three hours to maintain an even blood sugar level. (See "Hypoglycemia.")

Magnesium can also assuage the stressful symptoms of hyperactivity by strengthening the filtering device in the limbic system of the brain. If that system is not working optimally, too many extraneous stimuli are allowed to enter and find their way to the cortex, arousing the child to feel that action is required. Magnesium helps suppress the arousal potential of these unimportant stimuli at their source. A good dosage is 500 milligrams daily.

Unhappy Skater's Stress Relieved

A mother sought help for her eleven-year-old daughter, who was an accomplished ice skater. Her parents put pressure on her to do well, and she put added pressure on herself. She wasn't sleeping well at night and was getting frequent colds. In a private conversation with one of the authors, she spoke of how unhappy she was and how she had no time for a normal life. But she dared not tell her parents, who had spent a great deal of money on her skating lessons and uniforms.

A consultation with the parents revealed that they had no idea their daughter felt so pressured. They agreed that she could take one or two days off each week. Her skating coach was not pleased, but the sense of control the girl got from choosing what she wanted to do on her days off made all the difference in her sense of well-being. Skullcap Oats helped calm her so she could sleep at night, and Rescue Remedy eased her stress level; but just getting some time of her own may have done her more good than anything else.

STUTTERING (See Speech Development)

STYE (See Eye Infection)

SUDDEN INFANT DEATH SYNDROME (SIDS)

SUDDEN INFANT death syndrome, or crib death, strikes two out of every thousand babies at age two to six months and accounts for almost 40 percent of the total infant mortality. The baby is found dead in his crib, but postmortem examination can find no explanation. Proposed possibilities include sudden pneumonia, septicemia (blood poisoning), intracranial bleeding, low gamma globulin (blood proteins that fight infection), deranged calcium metabolism, partial dislocation of the top of the cervical vertebrae pressing on the brain stem, and a narrowed passageway at the back of the nose; but none of these factors has been found consistently in cases of SIDS.

Another suspected link is with infant immunizations, especially the DPT shot. Periods of irregular breathing and spells of apnea (cessation of breathing) have been documented beginning on the first day after these shots.[209] Since the age of vulnerability to SIDS is from two to six months of age, it seems prudent to wait until after that time for the shots if they are elected.

An increased incidence of SIDS has also been reported for babies who sleep on their stomachs. Government-mandated fire retardants in mattress covers contain phosphorus or an arsenic-based chemical. The warm, moist air from the baby in the prone position is thought to turn the chemicals into lethal phosphine or arsine gases.[210] Toxins from household fungi may compound the problem; so may vaccinations, which can cause fever and a more rapid, hot breath from the baby, enhancing the production of toxic gases from the mattress cover. In New Zealand, the incidence of SIDS dropped to zero over a five-year period with the use of mattress covers not treated with these chemicals.[211]

A correlation has also been observed between the number of silver/mercury amalgam fillings in the mothers' teeth and the amount of mercury found in the brain tissue of babies dying from unknown causes.[212]

Medical researcher Joseph G. Hattersley of Olympia, Washington, suggests that heart attacks may be the cause of SIDS. Cow's milk contains several times more methionine than human milk. Methionine is the source of homocysteine, which generates oxysterols, the source of the fatty material in the blood vessels contributing to heart attacks. SIDS is virtually unknown in underdeveloped countries living on traditional diets low in animal proteins. Vitamins C and vitamin B$_6$ have been found to be protective against the toxic homocysteine that comes from a high-animal-protein diet.[213]

SUNBURN, SKIN CANCER, SUNSCREEN HAZARDS, RICKETS

AT ONE time, the medical profession promoted sunbathing as beneficial for children. Ancient cultures venerated the sun as a source of life. Later, science discovered the relationship between vitamin D and sunlight, and between vitamin D deficiency and childhood rickets. In 1903, Niels Finsen was awarded a Nobel Prize for his Finsen light therapy for infectious diseases, and suntanning became a fad. Then an epidemic of skin cancer was observed in the 1970s (generally blamed on the thinning of the ozone layer), and the pendulum swung back the other way.[214] Pediatricians today tend to recommend dosing children with sunblock at every opportunity.

Despite these preventive measures, one out of six Americans can now expect to contract skin cancer, which is by far the most common cancer in the world. Fortunately, most cases are easily curable. At one time, these conditions weren't even classified as cancers for statistical purposes. (Skeptical statisticians suggest the classification was changed to improve the cancer "cure rate" from conventional treatment.) The dangerous skin cancers are the 10 percent that are melanomas, which progress faster than other skin cancers. Malignant melanomas can spread beyond the skin and are life-threatening. They are easily recognizable and are curable too, but they need to be detected early. **Suspicious growths should be examined by a dermatologist.**

The Sunscreen Controversy

SUNSCREENS COME with their own hazards. They interfere with the synthesis of vitamin D, which is essential for strong bones; they contain toxic chemicals like titanium; and they give a false sense of security and encourage long periods in the sun. A study reported in the *Journal of the National Cancer Institute* in 1998 linked the use of sunscreens to an *increased* risk of melanoma.[215] Most sunscreens, regardless of advertising claims, block out only UVB wavelengths, not the deeper-penetrating UVA wavelengths. That the skin's surface doesn't burn doesn't mean it's not being exposed to harmful rays. The melanin produced on the skin by unblocked sunshine (the suntan) is what actually protects the tissues beneath.[216] Other studies have found that sunbathing that does not involve blistering actually protects against melanoma. Moderation and gradual adaptation to the sun appear to be the keys to safe exposure.[217]

Natural Prevention and Treatment

THE PRUDENT approach to sunbathing is to build up exposure gradually—just to the point of a slight pinkish capillary dilation. This allows tolerance and still affords protection from vitamin D deficiency. Research has shown that even minimal exposure to blue sky is sufficient to prevent rickets. If longer sun exposure can't be avoided, protect your child with lightweight, light-colored, long-sleeved clothing and brimmed hats. If you need sunscreens, natural sunscreens without harmful chemical additives and preservatives are available at health food stores. Those containing PABA (para-amino benzoic acid) should be avoided. A recent FDA report concluded that fourteen out of seventeen suntan lotions containing PABA could be carcinogenic.[218]

Zane Kime, M.D., in a groundbreaking book called *Sunlight,* demonstrated that the sun creates free radical damage to the skin only in the absence of protective antioxidants and the presence of harmful fats. The antioxidants he discussed were vitamins A, C, and E and the trace mineral selenium, but there are many others. Harmful fats include hydrogenated oils, refined oils, and saturated fat; i.e., the fats in the standard American high-fat diet.[219]

 Natural Sunburn Relief

IF YOUR child has gotten sunburned, natural remedies are available to relieve pain and speed healing. Aloe vera has produced amazing results, especially with the fresh plant. The procedure is to simply cut open the plant and apply it directly to the burn. Aloe vera has been known to heal even severe burns in just a day or two when applied immediately.

Homeopathic Cantharis and Causticum are other effective remedies for burns and sunburn.

An old-fashioned early-stage remedy is to pat the sunburn with apple cider vinegar. It changes the pH and diminishes the sting.

Zinc has been shown to improve healing time from sunburn.

SURGICAL TRAUMA

SURGERY REPRESENTS a major stress to the body, and anesthetics and painkillers impose a sluggish drain on nerve and circulatory energy. A fundamental principle of Chinese medicine is that the body is criss-crossed with "meridians," or lines of energy, which provide the vitality necessary not only for healing but to maintain the workings of the body. Surgery inevitably cuts through these meridians, blocking both healing and bodily function. Yet for children as well as adults, some-times surgery cannot be avoided. In these cases, natural remedies can minimize the damage and help speed recovery time.

Conventional Postsurgical Treatment

FOR POSTSURGICAL pain and trauma, the medical approach is narcotic analgesics that work by drugging the nerves. Morphine, codeine, and opium are narcotics that are natural plant derivatives. Synthetic or semisynthetic narcotics include propoxyphene (Darvon), meperidine (Demerol), pentazocine (Talwin), oxycodone (contained in Percodan with aspirin and in Percocet with acetaminophen), and codeine (also used in cough medicines and for diarrhea). All narcotics can be addictive and have other side effects, including a weakening of the body's immune defenses. Anesthetics also linger in the system and suppress its functioning. If the system can't eliminate the drugs, the patient will continue to feel dragged out, tired, and sluggish.

 ## Aiding Recovery with Homeopathic Remedies

HOMEOPATHIC REMEDIES can cut the amount of narcotic analgesics needed after surgery, and they can alleviate the physical effects of shock. The best time to begin giving homeopathic remedies for surgical trauma is when the child is being wheeled into the operating room. Since they are taken sublingually (under the tongue), they won't create nausea or vomiting, as food will if taken immediately before anesthesia. The remedies may all be mixed and taken at once.

Aconitum is a common homeopathic remedy for sudden and violent onset of shock or trauma and for fear and anxiety, such as before surgery. In one double-blind randomized trial involving fifty children undergoing surgery, a significant reduction in postoperative pain and agitation was experienced by those given this homeopathic remedy.[220] If your child must undergo surgery, give Aconitum 6c or 30c the night before the operation and again in the morning on awakening, to help keep the body from going into shock. If anxiety continues after surgery, give one to three more doses.

Homeopathic remedies can also speed recovery and healing after surgery and reduce postsurgical pain and bruising. Recommended remedies include:

1. Arnica, to stop the body from overreacting to trauma. Give a couple of pellets of Arnica 200c when the child is being wheeled into the operating room, then four hours later. If needed, Arnica 30c may be given for several days thereafter. After the Arnica has done its job—that is, once the patient is free of pain—it isn't needed anymore.

2. Ledum helps to heal injuries that result in bruising and puffy skin, as first aid, to prevent infection, and for eye injuries. It should be taken in the same way as homeopathic Arnica, but after the second or third day, it can usually be discontinued.

3. Bellis is used to relieve blunt pain or trauma (the feeling of being hit in the face or of breaking the nose), to speed recovery after surgery, to help prevent infection, to treat abscesses, and to reduce swelling.

4. Calendula helps with wounds that are slow to heal.

5. Hypericum is used as a tonic for the nervous system and kidneys, and to treat puncture wounds and pain after dental work. After surgery, it is particularly useful for treating pain caused by injury to the nerve endings.

6. Phosphorus is used to treat anxiety, nervous and digestive ills, and respiratory and circulatory problems. In conjunction with surgical procedures, Phosphorus 6c or 30c helps relieve bleeding, nausea, and the lingering effects of anesthetics.

7. Staphysagria aids in relieving the pain of incision. Staphysagria 30c may be taken four times a day following surgery, until pain-free.

8. Cantharis is useful in conjunction with surgery for reducing the redness and swelling of burns.

Preparing for Surgery: Nutritional and Psychological Support

SUPPORT THE body's attempt to heal itself with nutritional and herbal supplements, proper diet, and toning exercises. Additional vitamin C, vitamin B$_6$, and magnesium are particularly important. Stress can exhaust nutritional stores and weaken the body's ability to recover. The state of mind in which surgery is entered into is also important. Try to reassure and calm your child so that he or she goes into the operating room in a positive and relaxed frame of mind. A few drops of Rescue Remedy, a Bach flower remedy, can help relax the child.

 Recovery from Surgical Scars

FOR SPEEDING the healing of surgical scars, a remedy called ScarGo by Home Health, containing olive oil, peanut oil, lanolin, camphor, and yellow beeswax, does a remarkable job.

SWIMMER'S EAR (See Fungal Infections)

TEAR-DUCT OBSTRUCTION (See Nasolacrimal Duct Obstruction)

TEETHING (See Dental Problems)

TEMPER TANTRUMS (See Anger)

TEMPOROMANDIBULAR JOINT DYSFUNCTION (See Dental Problems)

THUMB SUCKING (See Nail Biting)

THRUSH (See Candidiasis)

THYROID, HYPO- AND HYPER- (See Hypothyroidism, Hyperthyroidism)

TICK BITES (See Lyme Disease)

TICS, TOURETTE'S SYNDROME

TICS ARE spasms of muscle groups that appear to be involuntary, although if the child "really tries," he can reduce their repetitive frequency. Blinking, turning the head, shrugging the shoulders, and wrinkling the forehead are all common. The child is frequently tense and perfectionistic, as if he is trying to control the need to shout, jump, or run—bottled-up tension that is released in the tic. Most tics are considered developmental disorders. They typically appear when school starts, and in 80 percent of cases they disappear completely by about eight years of age. Tics are assumed to be a neurotic expression, but some violent tics may be associated with an epileptic disturbance, Tourette's syndrome, or other disease of or injury to the nervous system.

Tourette's syndrome is a neurological disorder characterized by repeated involuntary movements (tics) and uncontrollable vocal sounds, sometimes involving cursing and other inappropriate language. The child appears "possessed" or seems to have two personalities. The condition is considered genetic but has also been linked to certain drugs, including amphetamines and anti-psychotics.

Tourette's Syndrome Alleviated without Drugs

An eleven-year-old boy was brought to author Dr. Walker by his grandmother. She said the boy's parents were reluctant to come because they had been persuaded his condition was hopeless, but they were at their wits' end. The boy suffered from tics about fifty times daily, along with obsessive behavior that was out of control. The first two homeopathic remedies Dr. Walker tried made no difference at all. Then she spoke at length to the grandmother. The key to the case proved to be that the boy behaved like two different people. One minute he was bright, helpful, and eager to please. The next minute he was mean, hateful, and intent on getting his way—and those were the times his tics and obsessive behavior were at their worst. Dr. Walker recommended Anacardium (a remedy appropriate for his specific symptoms and personality type). A huge change in his condition was evident after only two doses. He became happier and the tics dropped from fifty a day to only one or two a week.

 ## Conventional Treatment

THERE IS no conventional cure. For Tourette's, drugs may be prescribed to control symptoms, but they can have long-term side effects and are controversial. Neurological development should be checked by a doctor.

Natural Alternatives

IF NERVOUS tics develop after school starts, the child might be under too much pressure at school. Some sensitive children do better with homeschooling. Parents should not scold children for tics or make them self-conscious about them, as the child wants the affliction no more than the parent does.

Homeopathic remedies, including Nat mur and Agaricus, may help relieve symptoms. Magnesium may also help.

TINNITUS (See Hearing Impairment)

TMJ (TEMPOROMANDIBULAR JOINT) DYSFUNCTION (See Dental Problems)

TOILET TRAINING

DECADES AGO, pediatricians believed that babies could be encouraged to "establish the habit" at about ten months of age. The recommended protocol was to simply place them on the toilet after breakfast when that unmistakable expression appeared on their faces indicating the rectum was about to empty. The ploy worked for a few cooperative children, but it also tended to make them obsessive-compulsive string-saver types; and it didn't work for the majority. Although bowel and bladder control is eagerly sought by parents as a sign of maturity and obedience in their children, when energy is applied too early or too forcefully to this goal, success is generally delayed.

The rule is that the older the child, the shorter the training period. "Learning waits on maturation" is a developmental truism. The infant controls his head when the nerves to the neck muscles mature. He can sit well by ten months, when the nerves to the back muscles have matured. Walking is possible at twelve to fifteen months, when the nerves to the legs are fully myelinated and mature. The nerves to the sphincter muscles of the bladder and anus are the last to mature. Forcing bowel training or getting upset with a child before these connections are made is counterproductive, promotes a bad self-image, and does not train the child.

Maturation varies among children and between sexes. Girls seem to become aware of the issue and want to defecate in the toilet by about two years of age, while boys may be ready only by three years of age. A sensible approach is to wait until the child is two years old, then dress him or her in training pants with a diaper inside and a plastic liner outside, an arrangement that is easy to pull off when the urge strikes. The Tom Sawyer ploy for whitewashing the fence sometimes works: The parent demonstrates the procedure, remarks on how good it feels, and hopes the child will want to imitate it.

Control over urination comes later than bowel control and is rare even during the daytime under eighteen months of age. Parents should expect some dry periods of two to three hours once walking has been mastered, usually after fifteen to eighteen months of age. Unfortunately, that is also the time when the child is likely to start asserting his independence and saying "no," and the game of wills begins. If a child has not passed beyond his infantile automatic involuntary bladder-emptying by the age of two (that is, if there are not an increasing number of dry periods), have your doctor investigate the urinary system to rule out possible organic causes. These could include a narrowing of part of the urethra, bladder infection (cystitis), a congenitally small bladder, a "nervous" bladder (the child who urinates when excited—something for which magnesium can help), or a sensitivity to some food (milk, fruit, chocolate). For natural remedies, see "Bed-wetting," "Bladder Infection."

TONGUE BITE

TONGUE BITES are common in children, whose play results in many falls. When a child falls while talking, his or her teeth are liable to bite into the tongue. Because the tongue is filled with vascular tissue, bleeding can be profuse enough to alarm parents; but the plentiful blood supply to the tongue allows for rapid healing. Tongue bites rarely need suturing—a fact for which surgeons are grateful, since it is virtually impossible to get children to sit still for this procedure.

TONSILLITIS

TONSILLITIS IS an infection of the tonsils, a set of glands at the back of the throat. The adenoids may also be involved. At one time it was fashionable to remove these glands in cases of persistent infection, since they were believed to serve no important function; but this practice has declined. Naturopathic doctors view the tonsils as a first line of defense against disease. The tonsils serve to "catch" germs, keeping them localized in the throat area and preventing their spread through the body.[221]

 Natural Treatment

FOR CHILDREN with persistent and painful tonsillitis, homeopathic remedies can give relief. For a restless child with a sore throat, Belladonna is good. For a child with bad breath and a sore throat, Mercuris is the appropriate remedy. There is an effective Chinese patent remedy called Antiphlogistic Tablets for sore throat or tonsillitis accompanied by fever. For other remedies, see "Colds," "Strep Throat."

For children who get repeated attacks of sore throat or tonsillitis, try eliminating milk products (including cheese and ice cream) for a month to see if there is any improvement. Throat swelling can be caused by cow's-milk sensitivity. For milk substitutes, see "Nutrition."

Tonsillectomy Averted by Dietary Change

John, age ten, suffered from recurring strep throats. An ear, nose, and throat specialist advised surgical removal of the tonsils and adenoids. John's mother consulted with author Dr. Smith, who advised her to discontinue the dairy products in John's diet. The following year, John did not suffer from a single sore throat, and surgery was averted.

TOOTHACHE, TOOTH DECAY, TOOTH GRINDING, TOOTH INJURIES (See Dental Problems)

TOURETTE'S SYNDROME (See Tics)

TOXOPLASMOSIS

THIS DISEASE is caused by a protozoan parasite usually acquired from domestic cats, which carry the eggs in their stools. Humans may also become infected by ingesting poorly cooked meat. Toxoplasmosis can be acquired by an infant from the mother before birth, in which case the symptoms and signs usually become manifest in the first year or so of life. They can include visual impairment, learning disabilities, and mental retardation. There may also be a rash, swollen lymph nodes, an enlarged liver and spleen, an enlarged head, and seizures; and calcification may be noted in the brain upon x-ray. If toxoplasmosis is acquired after birth, it may be asymptomatic or have only mild symptoms, including generalized malaise, muscle aches, and swollen neck lymph nodes.

Caution: To avoid acquiring and transmitting toxoplasmosis, pregnant women should not change cat litter boxes.

 ### Conventional Treatment

THE DRUGS pyrimethamine and sulfadiazine are the standard treatments for children and adults; but treatment may extend for a year, and the drugs can cause serious blood disorders.

 ### Homeopathic Treatment

A HOMEOPATHIC remedy called Toxoplasmosis made by the German homeopathic company Staufen (available in the United States as series therapy from Deseret) can effectively relieve this ailment.

TRAUMA, BRUISES, INJURIES

MINOR TRAUMAS from household injuries are everyday occurrences with children. Conventional pain relief is with analgesics like aspirin or aceteminophen (Tylenol and others), but these drugs can have side effects and suppress what the body itself is trying to do. (See "Pain.")

 ### Natural Alternatives

NATURAL REMEDIES are available that can heal injuries and reduce trauma to the body without suppressing natural body functions. Homeopathic remedies work instead to encourage those functions. Arnica montana is one that can be highly effective for trauma. (Don't confuse homeopathic with nonhomeopathic Arnica, which is a poison and should never be applied to broken skin.)

Trauma by CompliMed contains Arnica along with Bellis for blunt trauma; Symphytum for broken bones; Rhus tox and Ruta Grav for muscle aches and pains; Calendula to promote healing; and Hypericum for nerve pain. It comes as a liquid and can be taken orally or applied topically to the injury. Other good topical homeopathic remedies for injuries include Trauma One by Nutrition Now and Traumeel by Heel, available as either topical creams or oral tablets and drops.

TRICHINOSIS (See Parasites)

TRICHOMONIASIS VAGINALIS
(See Vaginitis)

UNCONSCIOUSNESS (See Head Injury)

URETHRITIS (See Bladder Infection)

URINARY TRACT INFECTION
(See Bladder Infection)

VACCINE REACTIONS
(See Immunizations, Shock)

VAGINITIS, VAGINOSIS, VAGINAL YEAST INFECTION

VAGINAL INFLAMMATION (vaginitis) and vaginal infection are the most common gynecological disorders, prompting more than ten million doctor visits annually. Vaginal infections include:

* *Candidiasis* (yeast infection), a relatively harmless fungal infection caused by an overgrowth of yeast cells (candida). Symptoms include itching, burning, and a white discharge resembling cottage cheese.

* Vaginitis caused by bacteria (*bacterial vaginosis*). Bacteria are found naturally in the vagina, but this disorder results from a change in the balance of vaginal bacteria, as from antibiotics. The condition is characterized by a milk-like discharge with a fishy odor and can precipitate pelvic infection leading to infertility or complications of pregnancy.[222]

* *Trichomoniasis*, a sexually transmitted disease caused by a parasite. Affecting about 2.5 million women and girls yearly, it may have no symptoms or may involve vaginal itching, burning, and a yellow or creamy-white vaginal discharge with a strong odor. A mother affected with this infection during pregnancy may pass it on to her female baby at delivery. The presence of the infecting protozoa in a prepubertal child suggests the possibility of ongoing sexual abuse.

 Conventional Treatment

ANTIFUNGAL CREAMS like clotrimazole and miconazole were once available only by prescription but can now be purchased over the counter for vaginal infections. The National Vaginitis Association warns, however, that unless the sufferer has had yeast infections before and is sure of their symptoms, treatment should not be attempted without a diagnosis, since antifungals won't cure the bacterial and parasitic infections that have similar symptoms but more hazardous outcomes. For these, prescription medications are recommended. Recurrent yeast infections can be an indication of something more serious, like diabetes or HIV. The popular nonprescription antifungals can also have side effects, and the infection is liable to recur.

The usual treatment for trichomoniasis is with the antiparasitic drug metronidazole (Flagyl). However, the drug can have substantial side effects (see "Parasites"), and it is not completely effective; the infection is liable to recur. **Caution: Metronidazole is carcinogenic to rodents and should not be taken by pregnant women. Metronidazole taken with alcohol can result in nausea, vomiting, flushed skin, and difficult breathing.**

 Alternative Treatment

TO CORRECT overgrowths of yeast and other invaders, a proper acid-alkaline balance needs to be restored and maintained within the vagina. Yeast can't live in an acid environment. For an older girl, make a douche of acidophilus (one teaspoon of acidophilus powder in an ounce of water or milk) or apple cider vinegar (four tablespoons to one cup of water) to acidify the vaginal area. An herbal douche containing forty drops of echinacea, forty drops of goldenseal, forty drops of Calendula, and two tablespoons of aloe vera in a pint of water can also relieve symptoms. For a younger girl, add 1½ cups of salt and 1½ cups of apple cider vinegar to a warm half-filled bathtub. Have her soak for fifteen to twenty minutes once or twice a day for two to three days. A sitz bath containing Calendula and goldenseal can also soothe burning and itching.[223]

Garlic is known for its antifungal properties. In laboratory experiments, its antifungal activity has proved greater than that of the antifungal drugs nystatin and amphotericin B.[224] (See "Candidiasis.") Health food stores now sell deodorized garlic capsules that make this age-old remedy both easy to take and socially acceptable.

Other recommended supplements include vitamins A, E, C, and B_6, zinc, and grapefruit-seed extract. An herbal combination containing a mixture of powdered goldenseal, myrrh, and slippery elm may also help.[225]

To discourage vaginal yeast, omit foods from the diet on which yeast thrive. These include foods containing sugar, molds, or yeasts; and aged or fermented foods, including breads made with yeast, aged cheeses, vinegar, and beer. No anti-Candida diet will effect a permanent cure, however, unless the underlying problem is also corrected. See "Candidiasis," "Fungal Infections."

Good homeopathic remedies for vaginitis include Kreosotum, Cantharis, and Sulphur. A good combination hemeopathic remedy is Vaginitis by Hyland's.

For trichomoniasis, Staufen makes a safe, effective, nontoxic homeopathic remedy called Trichomonas Vaginitis. Comparable series therapy is available in the United States from Deseret. Use the remedy even with conventional treatment, to prevent future recurrences.

VISION PROBLEMS: ASTIGMATISM, CROSSED EYES, WALLEYES

ONE IN four children may have a visual problem that impairs learning, but the child himself may not know it. He assumes he sees what everyone else sees. If the problem goes unnoticed, he may wind up labeled a slow learner. Telltale signs of vision problems include squinting, covering one eye, excessive blinking, dislike of close work, jerky eye movements, short attention span, daydreaming, placing the head close to a book when reading, losing one's place when reading, headaches, nausea, clumsiness, turning or tilting the head, and avoidance of reading. All children should have their visual acuity checked before the age of four or five. Besides nearsightedness or farsightedness, the child may have astigmatism, crossed eyes, or walleyes.

Astigmatism is a failure of the cornea (the lens of the eye) to properly focus an image on the retina. The child with this condition may have to hold printed matter in an odd position or squint to see well. He may also have headaches. Correcting nutritional deficiencies can be of some benefit, but the underlying problem is a physical defect in the eyeball. See an optometrist for glasses.

Crossed eyes also need corrective measures. The two crossed messages confuse the brain, which reacts by suppressing the image coming from one of the eyes. The result is called "suppression blindness." Surgery is sometimes recommended but is a risky solution. Developmental optometrists are the first professionals who should be consulted for this problem. They can prescribe exercises and corrective glasses to help the eyes work together.

Walleyes are eyes that turn away from each other. Again, surgery is a risky solution. Vision therapy is a less invasive alternative that can create a functional and cosmetic result.

Proper eye development and improved night vision may be aided with the herb bilberry. For remedies for tired or irritated eyes, see "Eye Infection."

VOMITING (See Nausea)

WALKER HAZARDS (See Crawling)

WARTS

WARTS ARE the second most common skin complaint after acne. Caused by the human papilloma virus (HPV), they are mildly contagious and can be spread to other parts of the body. Common warts are small, hard, round, elevated lumps, usually found on the hands. *Plantar warts* appear on the soles of the feet, where the pressure of walking pushes them inward. Most people get warts at some time, but children and young adults are more susceptible than older adults. Most warts go away by themselves, but this may take awhile—months or even years.

 Conventional Treatment

FOR THE impatient, there are medical remedies. Over-the-counter options usually contain salicylic acid (the main ingredient in aspirin). More invasive treatments include freezing, burning, or cutting off the offending growth; but these treatments are painful and can lead to scarring.[226] They also don't prevent recurrences and may even encourage them. When one wart is burned or frozen off, three are liable to pop up in the same or a nearby location. Since the cause is a virus, the problem generally runs much deeper than the manifestation on the skin.

 Natural Alternatives

HOMEOPATHIC TREATMENT takes a bit longer than cutting or burning, but it is more effective over the long term. Even if the warts are being burned off, homeopathic remedies should accompany them. The immediate effect will be to make the warts reappear, but then the virus will be cleared from the system. Likely homeopathic possibilities include Thuja and Causticum. Constitutional remedies specific to the patient can be selected by a practitioner.

Hannah Kroeger (Kroeger Herb Shop) makes a homeopathic wart formula called Wart that is simple and effective. It should be used both orally (ten drops three times a day) and topically (one drop applied to the wart three times a day) for three to four weeks. If any change at all

---

Warts Cured with Natural Treatment

A mother sought help from author Dr. Walker for her eleven-year-old son, who had a huge wart on his foot. The mother had tried everything, including having the wart burned off, but it had grown back. A single course of Thuja caused the wart to vanish for good.

In a second case seen by Dr. Walker, a mother brought in her daughter, who was chronically afflicted with warts. Dr. Walker suggested the Kroeger homeopathic remedy, but the mother returned to report that it had only made the condition worse. In fact, there were now more than 150 warts on the child, including 40 or so on her bottom. Further questioning revealed that she had had warts since she was six months old, and that her father had insisted on having them burned off. Every few weeks the mother would take the child to the doctor, who would burn off the warts, which would then reappear. This explained the "homeopathic aggravation" brought on by the remedy. (See Introduction.) Homeopathic remedies act by "pushing out" warts that have been suppressed by burning. The result was an outbreak of warts all over the body. Along with the warts, the child had a long history of behavioral problems. After carefully studying the case, Dr. Walker gave her Medorrhinum. In the first month the child's behavioral problems got worse, but more than half the warts disappeared. Four months later, only four warts remained and her behavior was very much improved.

is seen in the wart, continue the remedy. Otherwise, the remedy probably is not going to work.

Other natural remedies for which success has been claimed include methionine (one gram orally four times a day) and colloidal silver drops (twice daily).

Warts can be covered with plain bandaging tape to soften them up. To help "cook out" the virus in plantar warts, soak the feet in hot water at 118 to 120 degrees (as hot as can be tolerated) for fifteen minutes twice a day.

Homeopathically, warts have also been linked to worms. For worm remedies, see "Parasites."

WHOOPING COUGH (PERTUSSIS)

WHOOPING COUGH, or pertussis, is a bacterial respiratory infection that typically lasts six weeks. Two weeks of a dry, irritating cough without fever, usually occurring at night, are followed by two weeks of "whooping": The child coughs and coughs in spasms until all his breath is exhaled, then inhales suddenly and deeply with a characteristic whoop. He may turn blue in the face, cough so hard that he breaks capillaries in the skin of his face, or vomit severely enough to cause dehydration, weight loss, or malnutrition. Secondary ear infection and bronchitis are common complications. In the last two weeks of the disease, the cough reverts to the dry, irritating cough of the initial stage.

 Pertussis Immunization: Pros and Cons

A VACCINE is routinely administered to children to prevent pertussis, but the DPT (diphtheria/pertussis/tetanus) immunization remains controversial, having been linked to serious side effects. (See "Immunization.") Worse, it has not proved as effective as hoped in protecting children from pertussis. The statistics from an outbreak in Cincinnati in 1993 showed that most of the children who came down with the disease had had a complete series of shots along with a booster.[227] While the incidence of pertussis has decreased, it had already begun declining in the 1930s before widespread use of the vaccine. The symptoms of whooping cough have also gotten less serious, and this seems to be true whether or not the sufferer was immunized.

 Natural Alternatives

THERE ARE several good homeopathic remedies that help relieve the symptoms of whooping cough and boost the immune system in fighting it. One called Pertussis is also recommended preventatively, to be taken when the disease is going around but has not actually been contracted by the child. Remedies that can help relieve symptoms once the disease has been contracted include homeopathic Sambucus (elderberry) and homeopathic Ipecac (for a child who is coughing enough to induce vomiting).

YEAST INFECTION
(See Vaginitis, Candidiasis)

Notes

1. B. Goldberg, "Pharmaceutical Drugs: Your Money AND Your Life," *Alternative Medicine* (March 2000): 8; A. Levin, "America's Real Drug Problem," *Healthfacts* (June 1, 1998).

2. A. Lange, "Homeopathy for Childhood Ear Infections," *Nutrition Science News* (October 1996): 40; A. Chambers, "Drugs Increasing Health-care Costs," *Getting the Most for Your Medical Dollar* (August 1, 1995).

3. See M. Castleman, *Nature's Cures* (Emmaus, Penn.: Rodale Press, Inc., 1996), 218–20.

4. Ibid.

5. I. Kirsch, et al., "Listening to Prozac but Hearing Placebo: A Meta-analysis of Antidepressant Medication," *Prevention & Treatment* (June 26, 1998) (see American Psychological Association website, www.journals.apa.org).

6. S. Bharija, et al., "Acetylsalicylic Acid May Induce a Lichenoid Eruption," *Dermatologica* 177:19 (1988).

7. S. Begley, "Don't Drink the Water?," *Newsweek* (February 5, 1990): 60–61.

8. S. Roan, "Sufferers of Acne, Beware: Pimples May Be Winning," *Los Angeles Times* (May 8, 1996).

9. A. Shalita, et al., "Isotretinoin Revisited," *Cutis* 42:1–19 (1988).

10. E. Lammer, et al., "Retinoic Acid Embryopathy," *New England Journal of Medicine* 313:837–41 (1985); F. Tornatore, "Anti-acne Medication and Depression," *Psychopharmacology Update* (May 1, 1996); A. Shalita, et al., op. cit.; H. Roenigk Jr.,

"Retinoids," *Cutis* 39:301–5 (1987). See D. Blanc, et al., "Eruptive Pyogenic Granulomas and Acne Fulminans in Two Siblings Treated with Isotretinoin," *Dermatologica* 177:16–18 (1988).

11. A. Shalita, et al., op. cit.

12. "What's the Connection Between Hormones and Skin?," *Pharmacy Times* (May 1989): 49–51.

13. P. Boyer, et al., "Can Hormone Therapy Save Your Skin?," *Prevention* (January 1, 1997).

14. J. Trowbridge, et al., *The Yeast Syndrome* (New York: Bantam Books, 1986), 301–20.

15. See D. Gates, et al., *The Body Ecology Diet* (Atlanta, Ga: B.E.D. Publications, 1993).

16. For other home cosmetic ideas, see T. Jeffries, "Healthy Hints for Looking Good . . . Naturally," *Health Quest* (February 28, 1995); and T. Moore, *Kitchen Cosmetics,* reviewed in *Health Quest* (March 31, 1994).

17. "Plagued by Cures," *The Economist* (November 22, 1997): 95.

18. N. Freundlich, "Health: Fight Sneezing—Without Snoozing," *Business Week* (April 7, 1997); D. Levy, "Allergy-Relief Alternatives to Seldane," *USA Today* (January 14, 1997); "Slow, and Then Too Slow; FDA Falls Short in Dealing with an Already Approved Drug," *Los Angeles Times* (January 15, 1997); *Drug Facts and Comparisons* (St. Louis: Facts and Comparisons, 1998), 1229.

19. N. Freundlich, op. cit.; K. Painter, "Allergy Shots Give Little Help in Asthma Battle," *USA Today* (January 30, 1997).

20. See G. Maleskey, "Stuffed Up? Try These Natural Remedies," *Prevention* (September 1984): 63–6.

21. F. Batmanghelidj, M.D., *Your Body's Many Cries for Water* (Falls Church, Va.: Global Health Solutions, 1995).

22. S. Squires, "Allergy Season Returns," *Washington Post Health* (April 18, 1989): 6–7.

23. See R. Mendelsohn, M.D., *How to Raise a Healthy Child in Spite of Your Doctor* (Chicago: Contemporary Books, Inc., 1984), 205–6; L. Moll, "The Link Between Food and Mood," *Vegetarian Times* (August 1986): 28–30; R. Wunderlich, M.D., et al., "Nourishing Your Hyperactive Child to Health," *Good Health* 2 (5):16–19 (1984).

24. H. Sampson, et al., "Natural History of Food Hypersensitivity in Children with Atopic Dermatitis," *Journal of Pediatrics* 115:23–7 (1989).

25. R. Henig, "Who Gets Allergies?," *Washington Post Health* (May 31, 1988): 15.

26. P. Rowan, "A Brief Introduction to Bulimia Nervosa," www.prioryhospital.co.uk.

27. S. Roan, "Dangerous Combinations," *Newsday* (January 14, 1997); G. Cowley, et al., "The Promise of Prozac," *Newsweek* (March 26, 1990): 38–41; G. Null, "Prozac, Eli Lilly and the FDA," *Townsend Letter for Doctors* (March 1993): 1 ff; "A Prozac Back- lash," *Newsweek* (April 1, 1991): 64–7.

28. See, e.g., D. Lindenberg, et al., "D, l-kavain in Comparison with Oxazepam in Anxiety Disorders. A Double-blind Study of Clinical Effectiveness," *Forschr Med.* 108:49–50, 53–4 (1990); T. Munte, et al., "Effects of Oxazepam and an Extract of Kava Roots (Piper Methysticum) on Event-Related Potentials in a Word Recognition Task," *Neuropsychobiology* 27:46–53 (1993).

29. G. Lewis, "An Alternative Approach to Premedication: Comparing Diazepam with Auriculotherapy and a Relaxation Method," *American Journal of Acupuncture* 15 (3):205–13 (1987).

30. M. Loes, M.D., "Oral Combination Enzyme Formula for Difficult to Treat Joint Dis- ease," *The Doctor's Prescription for Healthy Living,* vol. 2, no. 5, See J. Theodosakis, *Maximizing the Arthritis Cure* (New York: St. Martin's Press, 1998), 206–15.

31. See M. Stoddard, *The Deadly Deception* (Dallas, Tex.: Aspartame Consumer Safety Network, 1996); H. Roberts, "Reactions Attributed to Aspartame-containing Products: 551 Cases," *Journal of Applied Nutrition* 40:85–94 (1988); H. Roberts, *Sweet'ner Dearest: Bittersweet Vignettes About Aspartame (NutraSweet)* (West Palm Beach, Fla.: Sunshine Sentinel Press, 1989).

32. Reuters, "Research Shows Junk Food–Child Asthma Link," August 22, 2000.

33. S. Stolberg, "Inhalers Linked to Cataracts," *Daily News* (Los Angeles) (July 2, 1997): 20; W. Hines, "For Asthma Sufferers, an Encouraging View of Overcoming a Lifelong Disorder," *Washington Post Health* (April 18, 1989): 6; L. Thompson, "The Asthma Dilemma: With Better Treatment Available, Why Are More Patients Dying?," *Wash- ington Post Health* (August 25, 1987): 12–14; "The Baffling Rise in Asthma Deaths," *Newsweek* (May 22, 1989): 79.

34. Gay Hendricks, "Conscious Breathing" (Audio Cassette: Audio Renaissance, July 1997).

35. R. Walker, "Fungus May Be Linked to Lung Disease," *Call and Post* (Cleveland) (January 19, 1995).

36. "Research Shows Junk–Food–Child Asthma Link," op. cit.

37. See R. Roberts, et al., *An Alternative Approach* (New Canaan, Conn.: 1997); "Plagued by Cures," *The Economist* (November 22, 1997): 95.

38. K. Woznicki, "Asthma Now: A Public Health Threat," www.onhealth.webmd.com.

39. A. Buist, "Asthma Mortality: What Have We Learned?," *Journal of Allergy and Clinical Immunology;* B. Lanier, "Who Is Dying of Asthma and Why?," *Journal of Pediatrics* 115: 838–40 (1989).

40. Asthma Center in Association with the Scripps Clinic, Allergy, Asthma and Immunology Division, "Asthma," onhealth.webmd.com.

41. F. Foulart, "An Alternative Approach to Reversing Asthma," *Alternative and Complementary Therapies* 3 (3):179–82 (June 1997), citing R. Firshein, *Reversing Asthma: Reduce Your Medications with This Revolutionary New Program* (New York: Warner Books, 1996).

42. W. Lewis, *Medical Botany* (New York: John Wiley & Sons, 1977), vii.

43. S. Lingling, et al., "Effect of Needling Sensation Reaching the Site of Disease on the Results of Acupuncture Treatment of Bronchial Asthma," *Journal of Traditional Chinese Medicine* 9 (2):14–43 (1989).

44. R. Roberts, et al., op. cit.

45. F. Batmanghelidj, M.D., op. cit.

46. L. Sroufe, et al., "Treating Problem Children with Stimulant Drugs," *New England Journal of Medicine* 289 (8):407–13 (1973).

47. R. Henig, "Courts Enter the Hyperactivity Fray," *Washington Post Health* (March 15, 1988): 8.

48. R. Pear, "Proposal to Curb the Use of Drugs to Calm the Young," *New York Times* (March 20, 2000): A1.

49. Ibid.

50. A. Morgan, "Use of Stimulant Medications in Children," *American Family Practice* 38 (4):197–202 (1988); "Methylphenidate Revisited," *Medical Letter* 30 (765):51–52.

51. L. Moll, "The Link Between Food and Mood," *Vegetarian Times* (August 1986): 28–30; R. Wunderlich, M.D., et al., "Nourishing Your Hyperactive Child to Health," *Good Health* 2 (5):16–19 (1984); "Hay Fever's Far-reaching Effects," *U.S. Pharmacist* (August 1989): 22.

52. T. Klaber, "Is Ritalin Necessary? The Ritalin Report," *Alternative Medicine* (March 2000): 89; J. Challem, "Reading, Writing & Ritalin," *Great Life* (December 1999): 36–39.

53. J. Challem, op. cit.

54. R. Mendelsohn, M.D., op cit., 205–6; L. Moll, op. cit.; R. Wunderlich, op. cit.

55. M. Boris, et al., "Foods and Additives Are Common Causes of the Attention Deficit Hyperactive Disorder in Children," *Annals of Allergy* 72:462–8 (1994).

56. J. Challem, op. cit.

57. Burton Goldberg Group, *Alternative Medicine* (Puyallup, Wash.: Future Medicine Publishing, Inc., 1993), 540–5.

58. "Breastfeeding and Oral Health," www.floss.com (World of Dentistry Online).

59. American Academy of Pediatrics, *The Tribune* (August 1997).

60. S. Virtanen, et al., *Diabetes* 49:912–17 (2000); J. Ismach, *Physician's Weekly* 14(35) (September 15, 1997).

61. See W. Crook, M.D., *The Yeast Connection* (Jackson, Tenn.: Professional Books, 1985), 291–2.

62. K. Kemper, M.D., *The Holistic Pediatrician* (New York: HarperCollins, 1996), 161–4.

63. "Quelling Candida," *Nutrition Science News* 2 (5):236 (May 1997).

64. J. Specht, "Should You Give Your Child a Chicken Pox Vaccine?," *Gannett News Service* (March 8, 1996).

65. *Drug Facts and Comparisons* (St. Louis: Facts and Comparisons, 1998).

66. V. MacDonald, "Asthma Steroid Can Kill, Health Officials Admit," *Sunday Telegraph* (July 20, 1997).

67. "Acetaminophen Doesn't Help Chicken Pox Sufferers," *American Pharmacy* NS29 (11):13 (November 1989).

68. Z. Zakay-Rones, et al., "Inhibition of Several Strains of Influenza Virus in Vitro and Reduction of Symptoms by an Elderberry Extract (Sambucus Nigra L.) During an Outbreak of Influenza," *Journal of Alternative and Complementary Medicine* 1:361–9 (1995).

69. S. Fishkoff, "A Berry Good Idea to Cure the Flu," *Jerusalem Post* (January 19, 1996).

70. M. Walker, "Olive Leaf Extract," *Nutrition Science News* (January 1998): 18.

71. "Cold and Flus," www.tnp.com (The Natural Pharmacist).

72. "Late News on the Cold Front," *University of California, Berkeley Wellness Letter* 5:4–5 (1988).

73. A. Orfuss, "Cold Sore," *Colliers Encyclopedia CD-ROM* (February 28, 1996).

74. M. Chohaney, "Hold On! Try This for Colicky Baby," *Capital Times* (Madison, WI) (May 1, 1997): 3F.

75. J. Zand, et al., *Smarter Medicine for a Healthier Child* (Garden City Park, N.Y.: Avery Publishing Group, 1994), 160.

76. L. Tierney, ed., *Current Medical Diagnosis and Treatment* (Stamford, Conn: Appleton & Lange, 1997), 228.

77. G. Lockitch, "Selenium: Clinical Significance and Analytical Concepts," *Critical Reviews in Clinical Laboratory Sciences* 27 (6):483–541 (1989); S. Uden, et al., "Rationale for Antioxidant Therapy in Pancreatitis and Cystic Fibrosis," *Advances in Experimental Medicine and Biology* 264:555–72 (1990); E. Kauf, et al., "The Value of Selenotherapy in Patients with Mucoviscidosis," *Medizinische Klinik* 90 Suppl 1:41–5 (1995) (in German).

78. H. Gelb, D.M.D., *Killing Pain Without a Prescription* (New York: Harper & Row, 1980), 43–4.

79. J. Yiamouyiannis, *Fluoride: The Aging Factor* (Delaware, Ohio: Health Action Press, 1986).

80. J. Yiamouyiannis, "Water Fluoridation and Tooth Decay: Results from the 1986–1987 National Survey of U.S. Schoolchildren," *Fluoride* 23 (2):55–67 (1990).

81. E. Brown, R. Hansen, D.M.D., *The Key to Ultimate Health* (Fullerton, Calif.: Advanced Health Research Publishing, 1998).

82. W. Price, *Nutrition and Physical Degeneration* (New Canaan, Conn.; repub. 1989, Keats Publishing, Inc.), 377–8.

83. H. Hawkins, *Applied Nutrition* (La Habra, Calif.: International College of Applied Nutrition, 1947).

84. W. Price, op. cit., 288, 444–9.

85. J. Ott, *Health and Light* (Devin-Adair, 1972).

86. D. Kotulak, et al., *American Medical Association Complete Guide to Your Children's Health* (New York: Random House, 1999), 467–8.

87. S. Satel, J. Nelson, "Stimulants in the Treatment of Depression: A Critical Overview," *Journal of Clinical Psychiatry* 50 (7):241–9 (1989).

88. S. Roan, "Dangerous Combinations," *Newsday* (January 14, 1997); G. Cowley, et al., "The Promise of Prozac," *Newsweek* (March 26, 1990): 38–41; G. Null, "Prozac, Eli Lilly and the FDA," *Townsend Letter for Doctors* (March 1993): 1 ff; "A Prozac Backlash," *Newsweek* (April 1, 1991): 64–7.

89. D. Manders, "The Curious Continuing Ban of L-tryptophan: The Serotonin Connection," *Townsend Letter for Doctors* (October 1992): 880–1; Citizens for Health, "Prepare for the Worst: FDA Propaganda Ready to Barrage Media," *Townsend Letter for Doctors* (August/September 1993): 860–1.

90. "PMS? Let 'Em Eat Carbs," *Vegetarian Times* (March 1990): 7.

91. M. Shangold, "Exercise in the Menopausal Woman," *Obstetrics and Gynecology* 75:53S–8S (1990).

92. S. Miller, "A Natural Mood Booster," *Newsweek* (May 5, 1997): 74; C. Jones, "St.-John's-Wort Gets New Attention," *Nutrition Science News* (September 1997): 436.

93. R. Podell, "Inositol Found Effective for Depression and Panic-Anxiety," *NFM's Nutrition Science News* (October 1996): 18; W. Poldinger, et al., "A Functional-Dimensional Approach to Depression," *Psychopathology* 24:53–81 (1991).

94. A. Stoll, "Choline in the Treatment of Rapid-cycling Bipolar Disorder," *Biol. Psychiatry* 40:382–8 (1996).

95. See D. Zimmerman, *Essential Guide to Nonprescription Drugs* (New York: Harper & Row, 1983), 449–71.

96. J. McEnaney, "Herbal Concentrates, Extracts Way of the Future," *Filipino Reporter* (December 7, 1995).

97. R. Henig, "Beyond Insulin," *New York Times Magazine* (March 20, 1988): 50–1.

98. J. Ismach, "Diabetologists Are Getting All Churned Up Over Cow's Milk," *Physician's Weekly* 14(35) (September 15, 1997).

99. M. Broida, "Cow's Milk and Type 1 Diabetes," www.tnp.com.

100. J. Classen, M.D., "Vaccines Proven to Be Largest Cause of Insulin Dependent Diabetes in Children," www.vaccines.net; see J. Classen, "The Timing of Immunization Affects the Development of Diabetes in Rodents," *Autoimmunity* 24:137–45 (1996); J. Classen, et al., "The Timing of Pediatric Immunization and the Risk of Insulin-dependent Diabetes Mellitus," *Infectious Diseases in Clinical Practice* 6:449–54 (1997).

101. "Plagued by Cures," *The Economist* (November 22, 1997): 95.

102. E. Burch, "Diet & Supplements for Diabetes," www.allHealth.com.

103. J. Anderson, et al., "High-Carbohydrate, High-Fiber Diets for Insulin-Treated Men with Diabetes Mellitus," *American Journal of Clinical Nutrition* 32:2312–21 (1979).

104. L. Nicholson, "Focus on Fiber," *Center Post* 10 (9):1, 7 (1989). See E. Brown, *With the Grain* (New York: Carroll & Graf, 1990).

105. E. Burch, op. cit.

106. "Silymarin May Help in Diabetes," *Let's Live Nutrition Insights* (November 1997): 9.

107. Zane Kime, M.D., *Sunlight* (Penryn, Calif.: World Health Publications, 1980), 39–41, 58–62.

108. K. Kemper, op. cit., 161–6.

109. D. Kotulak, op. cit., 282–3.

110. See D. Zimmerman, *The Essential Guide to Nonprescription Drugs* (New York: Harper & Row, 1983), 237–49.

111. A. Levin, "Diarrhea in Infants and Young Kids: Oral Rehydration and Homeopathy," *Health Facts* (June 1, 1994).

112. B. Wood, "Apples for Diarrhea," *Pediatrics for Parents* (November 1, 1993).

113. B. Hunter, "Beneficial Bacteria (Bifidobacteria)," *Consumers' Research Magazine* (January 1, 1996).

114. The study involved eighty-one Nicaraguan children, aged six months to five years, who were randomly assigned to receive either a homeopathic remedy or a placebo. Those in the treatment group received one of eighteen different homeopathic remedies normally prescribed for acute diarrhea, depending on the child's specific symptoms and traits (a departure from the standard study, which requires uniform doses of a single treatment). The children were also given oral rehydration. A. Levin, op. cit.

115. R. Davis, E. Braun, *The Gift of Dyslexia: Why Some of the Smartest People Can't Read and How They Can Learn* (Perigree Books, 1997).

116. G. Gates, et al., "Effectiveness of Adenoidectomy and Tympanostomy Tubes in the Treatment of Chronic Otitis Media with Effusion," *New England Journal of Medicine* 317 (23):1444–51 (1987); W. Crook, "Pediatricians, Antibiotics, and Office Practice," *Pediatrics* 76 (1):139–40 (1985).

117. G. Gates, et al., op. cit.; J. Paradise, "Otitis Media in Infants and Children," *Pediatrics* 65 (5):917 (1980); J. Paradise, et al., "Adenoidectomy and Chronic Otitis Media," *New England Journal of Medicine* 318 (22):1470 (1988); P. Lorentzen, et al., "Treatment of Acute Suppurative Otitis Media," *Journal of Laryngology and Otology* 91:331–40 (1977).

118. G. Gates, et al., op. cit.; T. McGill, et al. "A Seven-Year-Old Japanese-American Boy with Persistent Right-Ear Drainage Despite Antibiotic Therapy," *New England Journal of Medicine* 316:1589–97 (1987). The widespread use of antibiotics for treating ear infections is based on only a handful of studies, and their results have been questioned. See, e.g., W. Crook, op. cit.; M. Diamant, et al., "Abuse and Timing of Use of Antibiotics in Acute Otitis Media," *Archives of Otolaryngology* 100:226–32 (1974).

119. *The Medical Advisor* (Alexandria, Va.: Time-Life Books, 1996), 641–42.

120. W. Crook, op. cit.

121. E. Mandel, et al., "Efficacy of Amoxicillin with and without Decongestant-Antihistamine for Otitis Media with Effusion in Children," *New England Journal of Medicine* 316(8):432–37 (1987).

122. M. Casselbrandt, et al., "Otitis Media with Effusion in Preschool Children," *Laryngoscope* 95:428–36 (1985); J. Lous, et al., "Epidemiology of Middle Ear Effusion and Tubal Dysfunction," *International Journal of Pediatric Otorhinolaryngoly* 3:303–17 (1981).

123. J. Francois, "Corticosteroid Glaucoma," *Metabolic Ophthalmology* 2:3–11 (1978); R. Mohan, et al., "Steroid Induced Glaucoma and Cataract," *Indian Journal of Ophthalmology* 37:13–16 (1989); J. Henahan, "Study Shows Link Between Facial Steroids, Secondary Glaucoma," *Ophthalmology Times* (October 1, 1993): 32.

124. M. Rumelt, "Blindness from Misuse of Over-the-counter Eye Medications," *Annals of Ophthalmology* 20:26–30 (1988).

125. F. Fraunfelder, et al., "Systemic Side Effects from Ophthalmic Timolol and Their Prevention," *Journal of Ocular Pharmacology* 3 (2):177–84 (1987).

126. J. Kruse, "Should Fever Be Treated?," *Washington Post Health* (March 7, 1989): 11; T. Rosenthal, et al., "Fever: What to Do and What Not to Do," *Postgraduate Medicine* 83 (8):75–84 (1988).

127. T. Rosenthal, et al., op. cit.; J. Kruse, op. cit.

128. See J. Dobowy, et al., "Inhibition of Postpyrogenic Increase of Phagocytic and Killing Activity of Neutrophils by Nonsteroid Anti-inflammatory Drugs," *Archivum Immunologiae et Therapiae Experimentalis* 36 (3):295–301 (1988); E. Kiester Jr., "A Little Fever Is Good for You," *Science* (November 1984): 168–73; T. Rosenthal, et al., op. cit.

129. "Acetaminophen Doesn't Help Chicken Pox Sufferers," *American Pharmacy* NS29 (11):13 (1989).

130. D. Jaffe, et al., "Antibiotic Administration to Treat Possible Occult Bacteremia in Febrile Children," *New England Journal of Medicine* 317 (19):1175–80 (1987).

131. J. Whitaker, M.D., "Getting the Jump on Colds and Flu," *Human Events* (December 16, 1996).

132. Ibid.

133. Z. Zakay-Rones, et al., op. cit.

134. S. Fishkoff, op. cit.

135. J. Ferley, et al., "A Controlled Evaluation of a Homoeopathic Preparation in the Treatment of Influenza-like Syndromes," *British Journal of Clinical Pharmacology* 27:329–35 (1989).

136. T. Held, "Girl Dies from E. Coli Complication," *Milwaukee Journal Sentinel* (July 29, 2000).

137. See J. Foulke, "How to Outsmart Dangerous E. Coli," *FDA Consumer* (January/February 1994).

138. P. Phillips, "New Drugs for the Nail Fungus Prevalent in Elderly," *JAMA* 276 (1):12–13 (July 3, 1996).

139. R. Wild, "A Skeptic's Guide to Sports Medicine," *Men's Health* (April 1, 1996).

140. Ibid.

141. See K. McAuliffe, "Healing Therapies for Kids," *Good Housekeeping* (October 1, 1997).

142. N. Regush, et al., "Migraine Killer," *Mother Jones* (September 19, 1995).

143. "Doctor Discovers Aspirin-free Headache Cure," *Vegetarian Times* (April 1987): 10.

144. J. Carper, "Can Herbs Heal You?," *USA Weekend* (July 13, 1997).

145. "The Natural Way to Get Relief," *Redbook* (February 1, 1996).

146. "Magnesium Boosts Energy, Helps Migraines," *Let's Live Nutrition Insights* (November 1977): 6.

147. "Feverfew," *Vegetarian Times* (November 1988): 15; J. Carper, op. cit.

148. E. Infante, "A New Fight Over Common Lice Drug," *USA Today* (September 13, 1994).

149. G. Gates, et al., op. cit.; J. Paradise, "Otitis Media in Infants and Children," *Pediatrics* 65 (5):917 (1980); J. Paradise, et al., "Adenoidectomy and Chronic Otitis Media," *New England Journal of Medicine* 318 (22):1470 (1988); P. Lorentzen, et al., op. cit.

150. See E. Brown, R. Hansen, *The Key to Ultimate Health* (La Mirada, Calif.: Advanced Health Research Publishing, 1998); E. Brown, L. Walker, *The Informed Consumer's Pharmacy* (New York: Carroll & Graf, 1990).

151. S. Ziff, et al., *Dental Mercury Detox* (Orlando, Fla.: Bio Probe, Inc.), 37–40.

152. Y. Omura, et al., *Acupuncture Electrotherapy Research* 21 (2):133–60 (1996).

153. G. Bushkin, et al., "ALA Fights Free Radical Damage," *Nutrition Science News* 2 (11):572 (November 1997).

154. D. Ullman, *The Consumer's Guide to Homeopathy* (New York: Dorling Kindersley, 1995), 56.

155. R. Peat, *Nutrition for Women* (Eugene, Ore.: Kenogen, 1981), 16–21.

156. J. Lee, "Osteoporosis Reversal: The Role of Progesterone," *International Clinical Nutrition Review* 10 (3):384–91 (1990).

157. B. Eskin, et al., "The Disease in Disguise," *Good Housekeeping* (April 1, 1995); J. Lippert, "The Disease Doctors Ignore," *Redbook* (August 1, 1994).

158. W. Crook, op. cit.

159. Ibid.

160. M. Walker, "Olive Leaf Extract," *Nutrition Science News* (January 1998): 18.

161. Z. Zakay-Rones, et al., op. cit.

162. S. Fishkoff, op. cit.

163. J. Lieberman, *Light: Medicine of the Future* (Santa Fe, N.M.: Bear & Company, 1991), 141–3.

164. J. Orient, "Risk vs. Benefits of Vaccinations," *Congressional Testimony* (August 3, 1999).

165. H. Buttram, M.D., "Measles-Mumps-Rubella (MMR) Vaccine as a Potential Cause of Encephalitis (Brain Inflammation) in Children," *Townsend Letter for Doctors* (December 1997):100.

166. "Plagued by Cures," *The Economist* (November 22, 1997): 95.

167. H. Buttram, op. cit.

168. J. West, "Images of Poliomyelitis: A Critique of Scientific Literature," *Townsend Letter for Doctors & Patients* (June 2000): 68.

169. "What's Worse . . . The Insect Bite or the Insect Repellant?," *Townsend Letter for Doctors & Patients* (July 1997): 154; "Insect Repellants," *Medical Letter* (May 19, 1989): 45–46; "Are Insect Repellants Safe?," *University of California, Berkeley Wellness Letter* (June 1988): 7; "Prevention and Treatment of Insect Stings," *Pharmacy Times* (April 1989): 33–8; C. O'Neill, "The Big Sting," *Washington Post Health* (June 28, 1988): 22.

170. K. Kemper, op. cit., 265–72.

171. See S. Gilbert, "Eight Drugstore Remedies That Can Make You Sick," *Redbook* (February 1, 1996).

172. T. Gossel, "OTC Relief of Itching," *U.S. Pharmacist* (July 1989): 33–40; P. Parish, *Medicines* (London: Penguin Books 1989), 270–2.

173. T. Gossel, op. cit.; D. Zimmerman, *Essential Guide to Nonprescription Drugs* (New York: Harper & Row, 1983), 449–71.

174. See A. Convery, "Home Health Remedies That Doctors Recommend," *Cosmopolitan* (November 1, 1996), citing Jonathan Wright, M.D., and herbalist Jude Williams.

175. A. Solof, M.D., et al., "Newborn Jaundice," Vineland Pediatrics, P.A., www.cyberenet.net/~upeds HomePage (1993).

176. B. Arnot, "The Lowdown on Lyme Disease," *Good Housekeeping* (June 1, 1995).

177. See Moskowitz, "The Case Against Immunizations," *Journal of the American Institute of Homeopathy* 76:7–25 (1983).

178. L. Vorhaus, "Infectious Mononucleosis," *Colliers Encyclopedia CD-ROM* (February 28, 1996); A. Rochell, "Chronic Fatigue Syndrome Is Still a Mystery," *Atlanta Journal and Constitution* (March 27, 1996).

179. "Myth: Carbonated Beverages Relieve Nausea," *University of California, Berkeley Wellness Letter* 3(4):8 (1987).

180. U.S. Senate Document No. 264, 74th Congress, 2nd Session, 1936.

181. A. Gilligan, "Honey Not Safe for Babies, Parents Told," *UK News Electronic Telegraph* (May 18, 1997).

182. J. Mercola, "Fruit Juice May Cause Restlessness in Infants," *Townsend Letter for Doctors & Patients* (January 2000): 25, citing *Archives of Pediatric and Adolescent Medicine* 153:1098–1102 (1999).

183. F. Batmanghelidj, M.D., op. cit.

184. C. Keller, et al., "Childhood Obesity: Measurement and Risk Assessment," *Pediatric Nursing* 22:494 (November 21, 1996).

185. J. Hoffman, "Are Kids Really Getting Fatter?," *Today's Parent* 17:24 (February 1, 2000).

186. S. Roan, "Are Drugs the Answer to Childhood Obesity?," *Los Angeles Times* (December 25, 2000): S1.

187. Ibid.

188. E. Bravo, "Phenylpropanolamine and Other Over-the-Counter Vasoactive Compounds," *Hypertension* 11 (Supp. II):II-7–II-10 (1988); R. Glick, et al., "Phenylpropanolamine: An Over-the-Counter Drug Causing Central Nervous System Vasculitis and Intracerebral Hemorrhage," *Neurosurgery* 20 (6):969–74 (1987).

189. Associated Press, "Ephedrine Crackdown" (June 2, 1997).

190. "FDA Evidence Too Weak to Restrict Ephedra, Report Says," CNN (August 4, 1999).

191. "Sweetener, Brain Tumors Linked?," *Atlanta Journal* (November 5, 1996); "Olestra: Just Say No," *University of California at Berkeley Wellness Letter* 12 (5):1–2 (1996).

192. E. Neus, "Got a Cold? Is There a Pill Safe to Take?" Gannett News Service (January 18, 1995).

193. "Magnesium Boosts Energy, Helps Migraines," *Let's Live Nutrition Insights* (November 1977): 6.

194. J. Barilla, "Natural Remedies Show Effectiveness," *Health News & Review* (June 1, 1995).

195. See D. Kotz, "How Safe Is Your Water?," *Good Housekeeping* (November 1, 1995); "Study Says 2 Million a Year Suffer Water-Borne Illness," *All Things Considered* (NPR) (July 17, 1994).

196. A. Gittleman, *Guess What Came to Dinner: Parasites and Your Health* (Garden City Park, N.Y.: Avery Publishing, 1993).

197. "Pneumonia," *Tennessee Tribune* (October 23, 1996).

198. Safe Kids of Georgia, "Preventing Childhood Poisoning," www.choa.org/safety/poison.

199. D. Williams, "The Forgotten Hormone," *Alternatives for the Health-Conscious Individual* 4 (6):41–6 (December 1991).

200. B. Goldin, et al., "Estrogen Excretion Patterns and Plasma Levels in Vegetarian and Omnivorous Women," *New England Journal of Medicine* 307:1542–47 (1982); "Less Fat, More Grain Can Ease Breast Pain," *Vegetarian Times* (May 1989): 11; "PMS? Let 'Em Eat Carbs," *Vegetarian Times* (March 1990):17.

201. D. Duston (AP), "Calcium Seems to Help Women Deal with PMS," *Brownsville Herald* (Texas) (September 3, 1991): 14; S. Thys-Jacobs, et al., "Calcium Supplementation in Premenstrual Syndrome, a Randomized Trial," *Journal of General Internal Medicine* 4:183–89 (1989).

202. A. Gaby, "Calcium and Premenstrual Syndrome," *Townsend Letter for Doctors* (October 1992): 810.

203. J. Zand, et al., *Smarter Medicine for a Healthier Child* (Garden City Park, N.Y.: Avery Publishing Group, 1994), 360.

204. K. Kemper, op.cit., 207–8.

205. R. Lasser, et al., "The Role of Intestinal Gas in Functional Abdominal Pain," *New England Journal of Medicine* 293:524–6 (1975); *Federal Register* 47:486 (January 5, 1982).

206. G. Gates, et al., "Effectiveness of Adenoidectomy and Tympanostomy Tubes in the Treatment of Chronic Otitis Media with Effusion," *New England Journal of Medicine* 317:1444–51 (1987).

207. A. Bisno, "Acute Rheumatic Fever: Forgotten But Not Gone," *New England Journal of Medicine* 316 (8):476–8 (1987).

208. D. Kotulak, op. cit., 342–3.

209. V. Scheibner, *Vaccination* (Maryborough, Australia: Australian Print Group, 1993).

210. N. Tobitz, "A Possible Explanation for Sudden Infant Death Syndrome," *Our Toxic Times* (University of Oregon, January 1995).

211. V. Scheibner, op. cit.; J. Hattersley, L. Smith, M.D., *Infant Survival Guide* (Petaluma, Calif.: Smart Publications, 2000).

212. G. Drasch, et al., "Mercury Burden of Human Fetal and Infant Tissues," *Pediatrics* 153 (8):607–10 (1994).

213. J. Hattersley, et al., op. cit. See M. Suzman, et al., "Long-Term Mortality of Cardiovascular Diseases in Middle-aged Men," *Journal of the American Medical Association* 266:1225–9 (1973).

214. H. Randle, "Suntanning: Differences in Perceptions Throughout History," *Mayo Clinic Proceedings* 72 (5):461–6 (1997).

215. P. Autier, et al., "Sunscreen Use, Wearing Clothes, and Number of Nevi in 6- to 7-year-old European Children," *Journal of the National Cancer Institute* 90 (24):1873–80 (1998).

216. D. Williams, "Is the Sunscreen Craze Actually Causing More Skin Cancer?," *Alternatives* (April 1993): 2.

217. P. Wolf, et al., "Phenotypic Markers, Sunlight-Related Factors and Sunscreen Use in Patients with Cutaneous Melanoma: An Austrian Case-Control Study," *Melanoma Research* 8 (4):370–8 (1998).

218. J. Lieberman, op. cit., 152–4, citing W. Allen, "Suspected Carcinogen Found in 14 of 17 Sunscreens," *St. Louis Post Dispatch* (March 9, 1989).

219. Z. Kime, M.D., *Sunlight,* op. cit.

220. D. Ullman, *The Consumer's Guide to Homeopathy* (New York: Dorling Kindersley, 1995), 344, n. 1.

221. S. Harrison, *Help Your Child with Homeopathy* (Garden City Park, N.Y.: Avery Publishing Group, 1996), 63–4.

222. A. Hardie, "Women Seek Irritation Relief—Now," *Atlanta Journal and Constitution* (April 24, 1997). For a free booklet, *Women's Guide to Vaginal Infections,* write the National Vaginitis Association, 117 S. Cook Street, Suite 315, Barrington, Illinois 60010.

223. See J. Zand, op. cit., 411–14.

224. W. Crook, M.D., op. cit., 291–2.

225. "Vaginal Yeast Infections," *National Women's Health Report* (May 1, 1995).

226. *The Medical Advisor,* op. cit., 872–3.

227. C. Christie, et al., "The 1993 Epidemic of Pertussis in Cincinnati," *New England Journal of Medicine* 331:16–21 (1994).

Index

G

H